The Homemade Herbal Apothecary Guide

180 Timeless Home Remedies
Rooted in Tradition to Naturally
Support Everyday Health

Rowan Ellis

DISCLAIMER

The information presented in this book is intended for **educational and informational purposes only** and should not be considered a substitute for professional medical advice, diagnosis, or treatment. The remedies and recipes provided are based on traditional uses and historical knowledge, and individual results may vary.

Always consult a qualified healthcare professional before trying any remedy, especially if you are pregnant, nursing, taking medications, or have a medical condition. Readers are encouraged to research and use their own judgment before attempting any remedies or recipes in this book.

Neither the author nor the publisher assumes liability or responsibility for any adverse effects, allergic reactions, or consequences resulting from the use or misuse of the information in this book. By reading this book, you agree to take full responsibility for your health decisions.

Copyright © 2025 Rowan Ellis. All rights reserved. No part of this book may be reproduced, distributed, or transmitted in any form or by any means, including photocopying, recording, or other electronic or mechanical methods, without the prior written permission of the publisher, except in the case of brief quotations used in reviews or other non-commercial uses permitted by copyright law.

Published by Evergreen Compass Books

Printed in the United States of America

First Edition: July 2025

CONTENTS

Welcome to Your Herbal Apothecary 7

Essential Herbs   10

Tools, Techniques, and Preparations 18

Digestive Health   24

PEPPERMINT TEA FOR INDIGESTION 25	TURMERIC ANTI-INFLAMMATORY PASTE 36
GINGER-LEMON DIGESTIVE TONIC 25	CINNAMON BLOOD SUGAR BALANCE TEA 36
CHAMOMILE ANTI-SPASM TEA 26	CALENDULA TEA 37
FENNEL SEED AFTER-MEAL BLEND 27	PLANTAIN SEED CONSTIPATION RELIEF 38
SLIPPERY ELM GRUEL FOR ACID REFLUX 28	BLACKBERRY LEAF ANTI-DIARRHEAL 39
DANDELION ROOT BITTER TINCTURE 29	GINGER HONEY FOR NAUSEA 40
MEADOWSWEET HEARTBURN RELIEF 30	LEMON BALM NERVOUS STOMACH TEA 41
CARAWAY-ANISE GAS RELIEF TEA 31	BURDOCK ROOT DETOX DECOCTION 42
MARSHMALLOW ROOT INFUSION 31	CHICORY COFFEE SUBSTITUTE 42
LICORICE ROOT ULCER SUPPORT 32	PAPAYA LEAF ENZYME TEA 43
GENTIAN APPETITE STIMULANT 33	CARDAMOM DIGESTIVE CORDIAL 44
MILK THISTLE LIVER SUPPORT TINCTURE 34	YELLOW DOCK IRON TONIC 45
ARTICHOKE LEAF DIGESTIVE TEA 35	

Respiratory and Immune Support   47

ELDERBERRY IMMUNE SYRUP 48	HOREHOUND COUGH DROPS 53
ECHINACEA COLD FIGHTER TINCTURE 49	EUCALYPTUS STEAM INHALATION 54
THYME COUGH SYRUP 50	ASTRAGALUS IMMUNE BROTH 55
MULLEIN LUNG TEA 51	FIRE CIDER TONIC 56
SAGE THROAT GARGLE 51	OREGANO OIL FLU FIGHTER 57
PINE NEEDLE VITAMIN C TEA 52	HYSSOP EXPECTORANT TEA 58

COLTSFOOT CHEST RUB	59	ANISE SEED CONGESTION TEA	65
ELECAMPANE ROOT BRONCHITIS RELIEF	60	FENUGREEK MUCUS THINNER	66
		LINDEN FLOWER FEVER TEA	67
GARLIC-HONEY IMMUNE BOOST	61	ONION POULTICE FOR CHEST	68
ROSEHIP VITAMIN C SYRUP	61	HORSERADISH SINUS CLEAR	68
NETTLE ALLERGY RELIEF TEA	62	LOBELIA ASTHMA SUPPORT	69
GOLDENSEAL SINUS RINSE	63		
WILD CHERRY BARK COUGH SYRUP	64		

Skin and External Support 71

CALENDULA SALVE	72	YARROW WOUND POWDER	85
COMFREY BRUISE BALM	73	BEESWAX LIP BALM	86
PLANTAIN DRAWING SALVE	74	OATMEAL ECZEMA BATH	87
ST. JOHN'S WORT NERVE OIL	75	TURMERIC FACE MASK	87
LAVENDER BURN SPRAY	76	ROSEMARY HAIR RINSE	88
TEA TREE ANTIFUNGAL CREAM	77	PEPPERMINT FOOT CREAM	89
CHICKWEED ITCH RELIEF	78	ELDER FLOWER EYE COMPRESS	90
ARNICA MUSCLE RUB	79	BURDOCK ACNE WASH	91
WITCH HAZEL ASTRINGENT	80	VIOLET LEAF POULTICE	92
ROSE HIP SEED OIL SERUM	81	CAYENNE WARMING SALVE	93
ALOE VERA SUNBURN GEL	82	LEMON BALM COLD SORE CREAM	94
CHAMOMILE BABY BALM	83	THYME ANTISEPTIC SPRAY	95
JEWELWEED POISON IVY WASH	84		

Stress, Sleep, and Mental Wellness 97

PASSIONFLOWER SLEEP TEA	98	CALIFORNIA POPPY SLEEP SYRUP	102
VALERIAN ROOT TINCTURE	98	CHAMOMILE BATH SALTS	103
LAVENDER PILLOW SPRAY	99	HOPS DREAM PILLOWS	104
SKULLCAP ANXIETY RELIEF	100	KAVA STRESS RELIEF TEA	105
ASHWAGANDHA ADAPTOGEN BLEND	101	MOTHERWORT HEART CALM	106
LEMON BALM MOOD TEA	102	CATNIP CHILDREN'S CALM TEA	106

WILD LETTUCE PAIN SLEEP AID	107	ROSE PETAL GRIEF TEA	112
BLUE VERVAIN TENSION TINCTURE	108	HAWTHORN HEART SUPPORT	113
MIMOSA FLOWER HAPPY TEA	109	WOOD BETONY HEADACHE RELIEF	114
RHODIOLA ENERGY TONIC	109	JASMINE MOOD LIFT OIL	115
HOLY BASIL STRESS TEA	110	NUTMEG SLEEP MILK	116
MAGNOLIA BARK ANXIETY RELIEF	111	DAMIANA MOOD ENHANCER	116
OAT STRAW NERVE FOOD	112		

Women's and Men's Health   118

RED RASPBERRY LEAF PREGNANCY TEA	119	WILD YAM CREAM	128
CRAMP BARK MENSTRUAL RELIEF	119	MOTHERWORT PMS RELIEF	129
DONG QUAI WOMEN'S TONIC	120	ROSE HIP PREGNANCY TEA	130
VITEX BERRY HORMONE BALANCE	121	SHATAVARI WOMEN'S REJUVENATIVE	131
BLACK COHOSH MENOPAUSE SUPPORT	122	CLARY SAGE HORMONE OIL	131
NETTLE IRON-RICH TEA	122	RED CLOVER MENOPAUSE TEA	132
LADY'S MANTLE HEAVY FLOW TEA	123	FENUGREEK MILK SUPPLY	133
SHEPHERD'S PURSE BLEEDING CONTROL	124	PYGEUM PROSTATE HEALTH	134
FENNEL NURSING TEA	125	HORNY GOAT WEED TONIC	134
SAW PALMETTO PROSTATE SUPPORT	125	BLUE COHOSH LABOR PREP	135
TRIBULUS MEN'S VITALITY	126	PARTRIDGE BERRY PREGNANCY SUPPORT	136
GINSENG ENERGY TONIC	127	CORN SILK URINARY HEALTH	137
MACA ROOT FERTILITY BLEND	128		

Pain and Inflammation   138

WILLOW BARK PAIN TEA	139	CAYENNE PAIN SALVE	143
TURMERIC GOLDEN MILK	139	WHITE WILLOW HEADACHE TEA	144
DEVIL'S CLAW JOINT RELIEF	140	CAT'S CLAW ARTHRITIS SUPPORT	145
GINGER COMPRESS	141	FEVERFEW MIGRAINE PREVENTION	146
BOSWELLIA ANTI-INFLAMMATORY	142	JAMAICA DOGWOOD NERVE PAIN	147
MEADOWSWEET PAIN TEA	143	CORYDALIS PAIN TINCTURE	147

PINE BARK JOINT SUPPORT	148
CELERY SEED GOUT RELIEF	149
BUTTERBUR MIGRAINE TEA	150
BIRCH BARK MUSCLE RUB	150
YUCCA JOINT TEA	151
CLOVE TOOTHACHE OIL	152
BLACK PEPPER WARMING OIL	153
FRANKINCENSE JOINT CREAM	153
ANGELICA CIRCULATION OIL	154
WILD YAM ANTISPASMODIC	155
KAVA MUSCLE RELAXER	156
BLUE COHOSH CRAMPING	157
WINTERGREEN PAIN OIL	157

Children's Gentle Herbs 159

CHAMOMILE TEETHING TEA	160
CATNIP COLIC RELIEF	160
ELDERFLOWER FEVER TEA	161
LEMON BALM TUMMY TEA	162
DILL SEED GRIPE WATER	163
CALENDULA DIAPER CREAM	163
MARSHMALLOW SORE THROAT POPS	164
OAT STRAW BATH	165
LAVENDER SLEEP DROPS	165
FENNEL HONEY COUGH SYRUP	166
SPEARMINT UPSET STOMACH	167
ROSE HIP IMMUNE GUMMIES	168
SLIPPERY ELM LOZENGES	168
ECHINACEA GLYCERITE	169
MULLEIN EAR Oil	170

Seasonal Wellness 171

SPRING DETOX TEA BLEND	171
SUMMER COOLING HIBISCUS DRINK	172
FALL IMMUNE BUILDING SOUP	173
WINTER WARMING CHAI	173
NETTLE SPRING TONIC	174
DANDELION SPRING BITTERS	175
PEPPERMINT SUMMER COOLER	176
ROSE HIP FALL SYRUP	176
GINGER WINTER TEA	177
CLEAVERS LYMPH CLEANSE	178
ELDER FLOWER SUMMER COLD TEA	179
ASTRAGALUS FALL PREVENTION	179
CINNAMON WINTER CIRCULATION	180
VIOLET SPRING SYRUP	181
FOUR THIEVES VINEGAR	182

Welcome to Your Herbal Apothecary

Picture this: It's 2 AM, your child has a nagging cough, and the pharmacy is closed. You quietly head to your kitchen, open a special cabinet, and prepare a jar of thyme syrup. For centuries, families have turned to simple, natural remedies like this to help soothe discomfort and promote rest. While every individual is different, these time-honored practices remind us of the power of nature and the wisdom passed down through the ages.

What is Herbalism?

Herbalism is the practice of working with plants to support general well-being and address everyday discomforts. It is widely regarded as one of humanity's oldest health traditions, with evidence of its use dating back over 60,000 years. Many modern pharmaceuticals, such as aspirin (inspired by willow bark) and digitalis (derived from foxglove), trace their origins to plants studied and used by traditional healers.

What sets herbalism apart is its focus on whole plants rather than isolated compounds. For example, while a vitamin C tablet provides a single nutrient, an orange offers vitamin C alongside fiber, bioflavonoids, and other nutrients that work together holistically. This approach has been valued for centuries and remains a way to explore the natural world's potential to support the body's innate processes.

In this guide, you'll find recipes inspired by time-tested traditions that incorporate plants like peppermint, chamomile, and ginger. These herbs have been historically associated with digestion, relaxation, and general comfort. However, it's important to remember that herbalism is not a replacement for modern medical care or professional guidance.

This book does not diagnose, treat, cure, or prevent any disease. Instead, it provides natural options for addressing life's everyday discomforts—such as minor headaches, sleepless nights, or seasonal sniffles—that may benefit from gentle, mindful approaches. Always consult a qualified healthcare professional before trying any new herbal preparations, especially if you are pregnant, nursing, taking medications, or managing an existing medical condition.

Why Create Your Own Apothecary

Have you ever stood in the pharmacy aisle, feeling overwhelmed by the sheer number of choices and labels filled with ingredients you can't pronounce? Creating your own apothecary allows you to take a proactive role in your wellness and feel confident about what's in the preparations you use—because you made them yourself.

Beyond the satisfaction of crafting your own remedies, there are practical benefits to having a home apothecary. For one, it can be a cost-effective way to explore herbal traditions. A small bag of dried chamomile flowers, for instance, can be used to create dozens of cups of tea, tinctures, bath soaks, or salves—all at a fraction of the cost of purchasing these items pre-made. By building a small, versatile herb collection over time, you can make thoughtful, handcrafted remedies to suit your family's needs.

Freshness is another benefit. Commercial herbal products often sit on store shelves for months or longer, potentially losing potency. When you create your own preparations, you know exactly when and how the herbs were harvested, dried, and stored. This level of control lets you work with herbs at their peak.

But perhaps the most rewarding aspect of building an apothecary is the connection it fosters—to the plants, to traditional wisdom, and to your health. There's something deeply meaningful about knowing you can walk into your kitchen, open a jar of dried peppermint, and blend a soothing tea for your family. It's not just about the remedies themselves—it's about becoming an active participant in your own wellness journey.

Having your own apothecary can also help you feel prepared for life's minor discomforts. If someone in your household wakes up with a sore throat, for example, you might already have sage for a gargle, honey and lemon for soothing, or marshmallow root for coating. While these preparations are not a substitute for professional medical care, they can offer gentle, natural support for everyday situations.

Safety First: Important Considerations

Before we dive into the fun stuff, let's talk safety. While the herbs in this book are generally recognized as safe and have been used for generations, respect and common sense go a long way.

First, the golden rule: **start low and go slow**. When trying any new herb, begin with a small amount to see how your body responds. What works beautifully for your neighbor might not suit you, and that's perfectly normal. We're all biochemically unique.

If you're pregnant, nursing, or taking prescription medications, extra caution is needed. Some herbs that are perfectly safe for general use can interfere with medications or aren't appropriate during pregnancy. When in doubt, **consult with a healthcare provider** who's knowledgeable about herbs. Many seemingly innocent herbs like licorice can affect blood pressure, while St. John's Wort can interfere with numerous medications.

Quality matters immensely. A remedy is only as good as its ingredients. Source your herbs from reputable suppliers who test for contaminants and provide fresh, properly stored materials. If wildcrafting (gathering from the wild), be absolutely certain of your plant identification and harvest from clean, unsprayed areas.

Know when to seek professional help. Herbs are wonderful for minor, self-limiting conditions, but they're not appropriate for serious or persistent problems. If symptoms worsen or don't improve within a reasonable time, see a healthcare provider. A cough that lasts three weeks isn't just a cough anymore—it needs professional evaluation.

Keep detailed records of what you make and use. Note the date, ingredients, and effects. This isn't just good practice; it helps you refine your approach and creates a valuable reference for your family's herbal journey.

Essential Herbs

Building your herbal apothecary is like stocking a pantry—you want versatile basics that can be used in a variety of ways. Just as you wouldn't fill your kitchen with exotic ingredients you'll only use once, the same principle applies here. The herbs in this chapter have been valued for generations and are commonly included in traditional herbal practices for their broad range of uses.

The Top 25 Must-Have Herbs

These herbs are staples in traditional herbal practices and have been cherished for their versatility, ease of use, and long-standing presence in kitchens and gardens. Each herb has a history of being used in various ways and can be incorporated into teas, salves, oils, tinctures, and more.

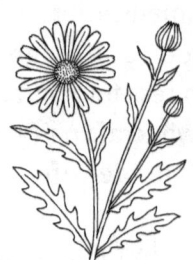

1. CALENDULA (*Calendula officinalis*)
Calendula flowers, with their cheerful orange hue, have been included in traditional herbal practices for skin support. They are often used in salves, oils, and baths. Historically, calendula has been associated with calming irritated skin and promoting cleanliness.

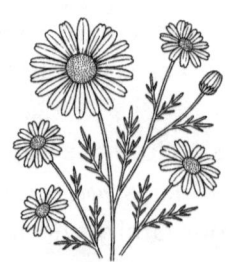

2. CHAMOMILE (*Matricaria chamomilla*)
Chamomile has been a staple of herbal traditions for centuries. Known for its gentle properties, it is often included in teas and preparations meant to promote relaxation. Chamomile is also commonly used to calm the digestive system. Its apple-like

scent makes it a favorite for teas, and it is mild enough for children when used appropriately.

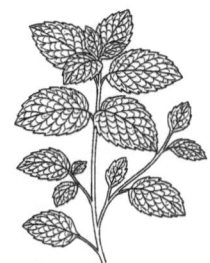

3. Peppermint (*Mentha piperita*)

Peppermint has a long history of use in traditional herbalism, particularly for digestive comfort and its cooling effect. It is often brewed into teas, made into balms, or added to steam inhalations for congestion. Peppermint is easy to grow, though it spreads quickly, so consider planting it in a container if space is limited.

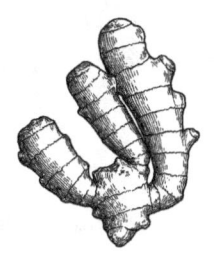

4. Ginger (*Zingiber officinale*)

Ginger has been widely valued across cultures for its warming properties. Traditionally, it has been included in preparations for nausea, digestive discomfort, and promoting circulation. Fresh ginger can be used to make teas or syrups, while dried ginger is often preferred in warming blends.

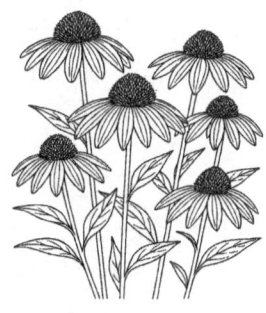

5. Echinacea (*Echinacea purpurea*)

This striking purple flower has been a favorite in traditional herbal practices for promoting seasonal wellness. While research suggests it may support immune function, echinacea is most commonly used at the onset of seasonal challenges. The whole plant—roots, leaves, flowers, and seeds—is often included in tinctures or teas.

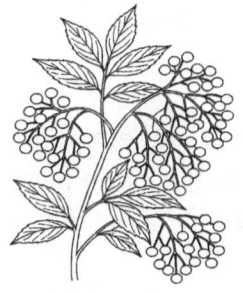

6. Elderberry (*Sambucus nigra*)

Elderberries have been cherished across generations for their use in syrups, teas, and other herbal preparations. Historically, they have been associated with supporting the body during seasonal ailments. However, raw elderberries must be cooked before use, as they contain compounds that can cause digestive discomfort.

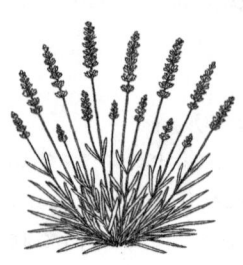

7. LAVENDER (*Lavandula angustifolia*)
Lavender's aromatic qualities have made it a favorite for centuries in herbal practices. It is often used in sachets, oils, or teas and has been traditionally included in preparations for relaxation and minor discomforts such as tension headaches.

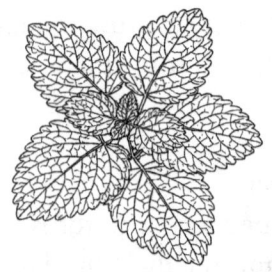

8. LEMON BALM (*Melissa officinalis*)
Lemon balm is a gently aromatic herb that has been traditionally used to lift the spirits and calm the mind. It has a mild, citrus-like flavor that makes it a favorite for teas, syrups, and tinctures. Historically, it has also been included in preparations for seasonal wellness.

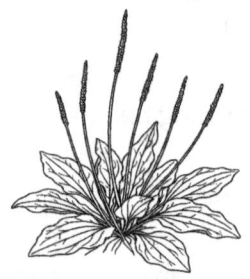

9. PLANTAIN (*Plantago major*)
This humble, often-overlooked plant has a long history in traditional herbalism as a "first-aid" herb. Fresh plantain leaves have been used for bug bites, minor cuts, and other skin irritations. Dried plantain can be infused into oils or made into salves for external use.

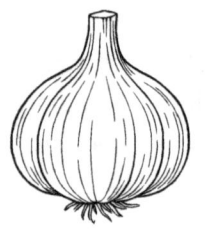

10. GARLIC (*Allium sativum*)
Garlic has been a cornerstone of traditional herbal practices. Often referred to as "kitchen medicine," garlic is commonly infused into oils, vinegars, or honey. Raw garlic is particularly potent, but cooked garlic still retains some properties.

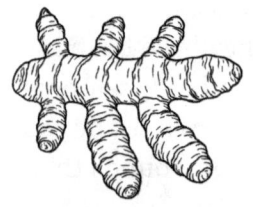

11. TURMERIC (*Curcuma longa*)
This golden root is a popular ingredient in both cooking and herbal traditions. It is often paired with black pepper in teas and other preparations to enhance its warming properties.

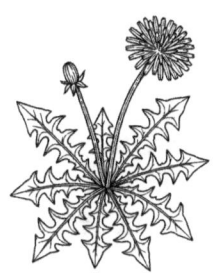
12. DANDELION (*Taraxacum officinale*)
Every part of the dandelion has been valued in traditional herbalism. The leaves are often included in teas or tinctures for their diuretic properties, the roots are associated with liver support, and the flowers are frequently infused into oils.

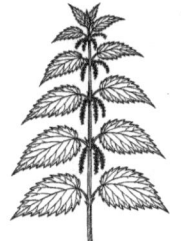
13. NETTLE (*Urtica dioica*)
Nettle is highly regarded in traditional herbalism as a mineral-rich herb. Once dried or cooked, it loses its sting and can be used in teas, soups, or broths. Nettle is often associated with seasonal wellness and nourishment.

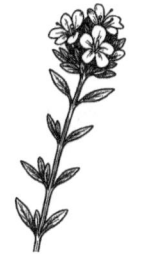
14. THYME (*Thymus vulgaris*)
Thyme is a versatile kitchen herb that has been traditionally used in preparations for respiratory support and general wellness. It is often infused into syrups, teas, and honey for its aromatic and warming qualities.

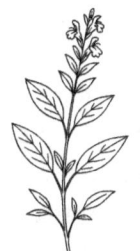
15. SAGE (*Salvia officinalis*)
Sage has a long history of use in herbal traditions, particularly for sore throats and digestive comfort. Its strong, earthy flavor makes it a popular choice for teas and gargles.

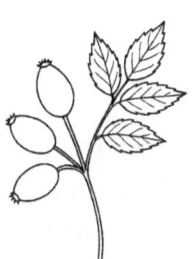
16. ROSE HIPS (*Rosa canina*)
Rose hips, often referred to as "nature's vitamin C source," have been traditionally used in teas and syrups for their tart, fruity flavor. They are commonly included in herbal preparations during the colder months due to their association with seasonal wellness. Harvest after the first frost for the best flavor, or purchase dried hips for convenience.

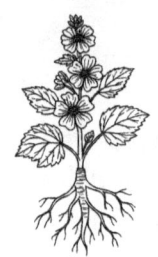

17. MARSHMALLOW ROOT (*Althaea officinalis*)
The marshmallow plant has been a part of traditional herbal practices for centuries, valued for its mucilage—a gel-like substance that coats and soothes. It has historically been used in teas or cold infusions for throat and digestive comfort.

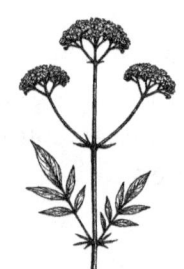

18. VALERIAN (*Valeriana officinalis*)
Valerian root has long been included in herbal traditions for its potential to promote relaxation. It is often made into teas, tinctures, or capsules, though its strong aroma may not appeal to everyone. Some individuals may find valerian stimulating, so it's wise to start with a small amount to see how your body responds.

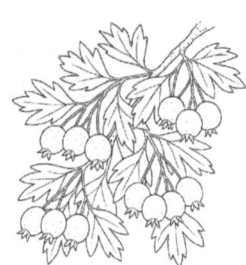

19. HAWTHORN (*Crataegus spp.*)
Hawthorn berries, leaves, and flowers have been cherished in herbal traditions for their association with heart health and overall well-being. Often used in teas or tinctures, hawthorn is considered a gentle herb suitable for long-term use.

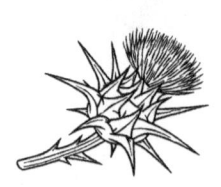

20. MILK THISTLE (*Silybum marianum*)
Milk thistle seeds have a long history of use in herbalism and are often associated with liver health. The seeds contain silymarin, a compound studied for its potential to support the liver. To use, grind fresh seeds and incorporate them into teas or tinctures.

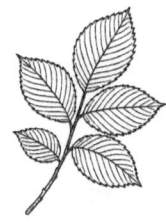

21. SLIPPERY ELM (*Ulmus rubra*)
Slippery elm bark powder has been traditionally used to create a soothing gel when mixed with water. This preparation is commonly included

in herbal practices for throat and digestive comfort. It can also be mixed with honey to make a lozenge-like paste.

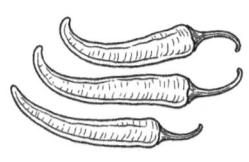

22. CAYENNE (*Capsicum annuum*)
Cayenne pepper has been a staple in both culinary and herbal traditions, valued for its warming and stimulating properties. A small amount of cayenne powder can be included in salves or liniments for external use, or in teas for internal warmth.

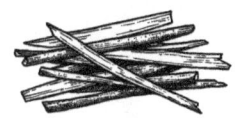

23. WILLOW BARK (*Salix alba*)
Willow bark has been historically used in herbal traditions for its salicin content, which is chemically similar to aspirin. It is often made into teas or tinctures and is most commonly associated with discomforts such as minor aches. However, individuals allergic to aspirin or salicylates should avoid willow bark.

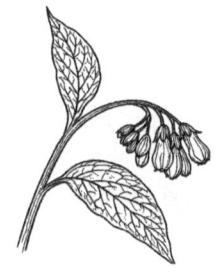

24. COMFREY (*Symphytum officinale*)
Known as "knitbone" in traditional herbalism, comfrey has been historically valued for external use in salves or poultices. It is commonly applied to bruises or minor injuries, but it should never be used internally due to the presence of compounds that may affect the liver.

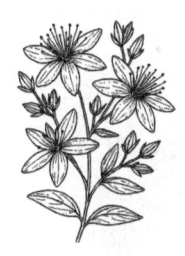

25. ST. JOHN'S WORT (*Hypericum perforatum*)
Sunshine in a bottle. The flowers make a beautiful red oil for nerve pain and a tincture for mild depression. Harvest flowers on a sunny day for best potency. Many medication interactions—research before using internally.

Where to Source Quality Herbs

Now that you know which herbs to stock, let's talk about finding them. Quality varies dramatically, and your remedies are only as good as your ingredients. Here's how to source herbs you can trust.

Start local when possible. Farmers' markets often have vendors selling dried herbs, and you can ask about their growing practices. Local herb shops let you see and smell before buying—trust your senses. Fresh, properly dried herbs have vibrant color and strong scent.

For online ordering, stick with reputable suppliers who specialize in medicinal herbs. Look for companies that provide harvest dates, country of origin, and organic certification. Good suppliers test for contaminants and store herbs properly.

When buying, consider these quality markers:
» Color should be vibrant, not faded or brown
» Scent should be characteristic and strong
» Texture should be appropriate—leaves crisp, roots hard
» No signs of mold, bugs, or excessive stems

Buy organic when possible, especially for herbs you'll use frequently. Pesticide residues concentrate when herbs are dried. For rare or expensive herbs, conventional might be your only option—just source from suppliers who test for contaminants.

Consider joining a community-supported herbalism program (CSH) if available in your area. Like CSAs for vegetables, you'll receive seasonal shares of locally grown herbs. It's a great way to try new herbs and support local growers.

Don't overlook ethnic markets! Asian groceries often have excellent prices on ginger, turmeric, and medicinal mushrooms. Latin markets carry many herbs like chamomile and hibiscus. Middle Eastern stores stock quality culinary herbs.

Growing vs. Buying: Making Smart Choices

The "grow or buy" decision depends on your space, time, and climate. Some herbs make perfect sense to grow, while others are better purchased. Let's be strategic about this.

ALWAYS GROW THESE:
- Lemon balm, peppermint, and other mints (they're invasive but easy)
- Calendula (self-seeds and blooms all season)
- Plantain (probably already in your yard)
- Thyme, sage, oregano (perennial in most climates)
- Chamomile (self-seeds readily)

These herbs are easy, prolific, and used frequently. Fresh is often superior to dried, and they'll save you money quickly.

USUALLY BETTER TO BUY:
- Roots like ginger and turmeric (unless you live in tropical zones)
- Tree barks like willow and slippery elm
- Exotic herbs outside your climate zone
- Herbs requiring special processing like elderberries
- Anything you use infrequently

CONSIDER YOUR REALITY:

A small balcony can support a surprising variety of potted herbs. Even a sunny windowsill grows decent amounts of essential herbs. But don't feel guilty about buying—purchased herbs are far better than no herbs at all.

If growing, start small. Choose five herbs you'll actually use rather than planting an overwhelming garden. Perennials give you the best return on investment. Group herbs by water needs—Mediterranean herbs like sage and thyme prefer dry conditions, while mints love moisture.

Harvest your homegrown herbs at peak potency: leaves before flowering, flowers when just opened, roots in fall or early spring. Dry them properly in small bundles away from direct sun, or use a dehydrator on low heat. Store in airtight containers away from light.

The beauty of combining growing and buying is flexibility. Grow what thrives in your space and brings you joy. Buy what's challenging to grow or process. There's no shame in purchasing herbs—traditional herbalists have always traded for what they couldn't grow locally.

Tools, Techniques, and Preparations

Think of this chapter as your herbal skills bootcamp. Just as a chef needs proper knives and techniques, an herbalist needs the right tools and know-how. The good news? You probably already own half of what you need, and the techniques are simpler than making Sunday dinner.

Essential Equipment and Storage

Let's start with the basics. Your great-grandmother made effective remedies with even less, so don't feel you need everything at once. Build your collection as you go.

THE NON-NEGOTIABLES:
- » Glass jars with tight lids (various sizes—save those jam jars!)
- » Fine mesh strainer or cheesecloth
- » Measuring cups and spoons (separate from cooking ones)
- » Sharp knife and cutting board
- » Labels and permanent marker
- » Small pot designated for herbs

THE NICE-TO-HAVES:
- » Mortar and pestle (granite or marble best)
- » Kitchen scale for precise measurements
- » French press (makes straining tinctures easy)
- » Herb press or potato ricer
- » Dark glass bottles for tinctures
- » Small funnel
- » Dedicated herb scissors

STORAGE WISDOM:

Light, heat, and air are the enemies of herb potency. Store dried herbs in airtight containers away from direct sunlight. That Pinterest-worthy open shelf with clear jars looks lovely but degrades your herbs quickly. Use amber jars or store clear jars in a cupboard.

Label everything with herb name and date. Trust me—dried green herbs look remarkably similar, and you will forget when you made that tincture. Include the moon phase if you're feeling witchy (some herbalists swear by it).

Whole herbs stay potent longer than ground. Buy or dry herbs whole, then grind as needed. Temperature matters. Store most preparations in cool, dark places. Refrigerate fresh preparations, oil infusions, and anything without alcohol preservation. Tinctures and vinegars can live happily in a cupboard for years.

Organization prevents overwhelm. Designate one cupboard or shelf for your apothecary. Group similar items: dried herbs together, tinctures in one spot, salves and oils nearby. When someone needs help, you can find remedies quickly.

Basic Preparation Methods

Now for the fun part—turning plants into herbal remedies! Each method extracts different properties and suits different purposes. Master these five basic preparations, and you can make 90% of the remedies in this book.

Teas and Infusions

The gateway preparation—if you can boil water, you can make herbal tea. But let's elevate your tea game beyond dunking a bag in hot water.

BASIC TEA: Use 1 teaspoon dried herb (or 2 teaspoons fresh) per cup of water. Pour boiling water over herbs, cover, and steep 5-10 minutes. Covering prevents aromatic oils from escaping. Strain and enjoy.

INFUSIONS: These are simply strong teas. Use 1 ounce dried herb to 1 quart boiling water. Steep covered for 4-8 hours or overnight. This method extracts minerals and deep nutrition from herbs like nettle and oat straw. Refrigerate and use within 48 hours.

DECOCTIONS: For tough plant parts like roots and barks. Use 1 ounce herb to 1 quart water. Simmer gently for 20-30 minutes, covered. The water should reduce by about half. Strain while hot. Perfect for roots like ginger and dandelion.

COLD INFUSIONS: Some herbs release their beneficial properties better in cold water. Marshmallow root is the classic example. Soak 1/4 cup root in 1 quart cold water overnight. The result is a soothing, mucilaginous liquid.

Pro tip: Make your teas in a French press for easy straining. Mason jars work great for infusions—the measurement marks are built in!

Tinctures and Extracts

Tinctures are herbs extracted in alcohol, creating concentrated, shelf-stable preparations. They're convenient, and last for years.

BASIC TINCTURE METHOD:
1. Fill jar 1/2 full with dried herbs (or 3/4 with fresh)
2. Cover completely with 80-100 proof alcohol
3. Label with herb, alcohol percentage, and date
4. Shake daily for 4-6 weeks
5. Strain, pressing herbs to extract all liquid
6. Store in dark bottles

GLYCERITES: For alcohol-free extracts, use vegetable glycerin. Mix 3 parts glycerin to 1 part water, then follow tincture method. These are perfect for children but less potent and shorter-lived than alcohol tinctures.

VINEGAR EXTRACTS: Use raw apple cider vinegar instead of alcohol. Excellent for mineral-rich herbs and culinary preparations. Fire cider is the famous example. Use plastic lids—vinegar corrodes metal.

The magic ratio for tinctures is roughly 1:5 for dried herbs (1 part herb to 5 parts alcohol by weight) or 1:2 for fresh. But don't stress—folk method (filling jars and covering) works fine for home use.

Salves and Balms

External preparations let herbs work their magic through skin. Once you make your first salve, you'll wonder why you ever bought them.

BASIC SALVE RECIPE:
1. Make herb-infused oil (see below)

2. Gently warm 1 cup oil with 1 ounce beeswax
3. Stir until wax melts completely
4. Pour into containers immediately
5. Let cool undisturbed

INFUSED OILS: The foundation of salves. Fill jar with dried herbs, cover with oil (olive, coconut, or sweet almond work well). For the slow method: let sit 4-6 weeks, shaking daily. For quick method: warm gently in a double boiler for 2-4 hours. Never let oil smoke or bubble.

CUSTOMIZING FIRMNESS: More beeswax makes harder salves, less makes softer. Cold climate? Use less wax. Hot climate? Use more. Test consistency by dropping a bit on a cold plate.

Add vitamin E oil (½ teaspoon per cup) to extend shelf life. Essential oils go in after removing from heat—about 20-30 drops per cup of oil.

Syrups and Honeys

Remedy that tastes like dessert? Yes, please! These preparations make herbs palatable for picky eaters and soothe throats while delivering beneficial properties.

BASIC SYRUP:
1. Make strong decoction (1 part herb to 2 parts water)
2. Strain and measure liquid
3. Add equal amount honey or sugar
4. Warm gently until dissolved
5. Add preservative (brandy or tincture) if desired
6. Bottle and refrigerate

HERBAL HONEY: Simply fill jar ¼ with dried herbs, cover with honey. Let infuse 2-4 weeks, warming gently if desired. Strain or leave herbs in. Rose petal honey is divine!

ELECTUARIES: These are powdered herbs mixed into honey or nut butter. Start with 1 part powder to 3 parts honey. Perfect for herbs that taste terrible—the honey masks bitterness.

Syrups keep 3-6 months refrigerated, longer with alcohol added (use ¼ part brandy to ¾ parts syrup). Herbal honeys last indefinitely if herbs were completely dry.

Dosage Guidelines and Administration

The million-dollar question: "How much do I take?" Unlike pharmaceuticals with rigid dosing, herbs offer flexibility. Your body often tells you what it needs.

GENERAL GUIDELINES:
- » Teas: 3-4 cups daily for acute issues, 1-2 for maintenance
- » Tinctures: 30-60 drops (½ to 1 teaspoon) 3x daily for adults
- » Syrups: 1 tablespoon 3-4x daily for acute issues
- » Salves: Apply as needed, usually 2-4x daily

ADJUST FOR BODY SIZE:
- » Children 50-75 lbs: ⅓ adult dose
- » Children 75-100 lbs: ½ adult dose
- » Over 100 lbs: ¾ to full adult dose
- » Elders often need less; start with ¾ dose

TIMING MATTERS:
- » Bitters: 15 minutes before meals
- » Digestive teas: with or right after meals
- » Sleep herbs: 30-60 minutes before bed
- » Immune herbs: throughout the day during illness

DURATION:
- » Acute issues: Take frequently until resolved (usually 3-7 days)
- » Chronic issues: Take regularly for 3-6 weeks, then reassess
- » Tonic herbs: Can take daily for months
- » Nutritive herbs: Safe for long-term daily use

LISTEN TO YOUR BODY:

Start with less than recommended and increase if needed. If an herb makes you feel worse, stop taking it—not every herb suits every person. Some people need double the standard dose; others are sensitive and need half.

DELIVERY METHODS:

» Empty stomach: Fastest absorption but might cause nausea
» With food: Gentler, better for long-term use
» In water: Dilutes alcohol tinctures for sensitive folks
» Topically: Great for local issues and those who can't take internally

Remember: more isn't always better. Herbs work gently to support your body's own healing. Give them time, be consistent, and pay attention to how you feel. Your body's wisdom, combined with nature's pharmacy, creates true healing.

Digestive Health

Your digestive system is like the roots of a tree—when it's healthy, the whole organism thrives. When it's struggling, nothing feels quite right. From that morning coffee rumble to after-dinner bloating, digestive complaints are among the most common reasons people turn to herbal remedies. The good news? Plants have been helping human digestion since we first learned to eat.

Understanding Digestive Wellness

Think of your digestive system as a long, winding river that transforms food into life. It begins in your mouth and ends... well, you know where. Along the way, this amazing system breaks down food, absorbs nutrients, houses most of your immune system, and even produces neurotransmitters that affect your mood.

When this river flows smoothly, you barely notice it's there. But when something creates a dam or disruption—stress, poor food choices, illness, medications—the whole system backs up. That's when you might experience heartburn creeping up your chest, bloating that makes your favorite jeans uncomfortable, or that anxious stomach that shows up before important meetings.

The herbs in this chapter work in different ways to support digestive flow. Some stimulate digestive juices (we call these bitters), others soothe inflammation, and some provide protective coatings to irritated tissues. Many work on multiple levels—chamomile, for instance, relaxes both smooth muscle spasms and the anxious mind that often triggers them.

Herbs for Digestive Issues

PEPPERMINT TEA FOR INDIGESTION

Ancient Greeks and Romans crowned themselves with peppermint at feasts, believing it prevented indigestion. They were onto something—peppermint remains one of our most reliable digestive aids.

What You'll Need:
» 2 tablespoons fresh peppermint leaves (or 1 tablespoon dried)
» 1 cup boiling water
» Honey to taste (optional)
» Fresh lemon slice (optional)

How to Make It:
1. Place peppermint leaves in a teapot or mug
2. Pour boiling water over the leaves
3. Cover and steep for 7-10 minutes
4. Strain out the leaves
5. Add honey and lemon if desired
6. Sip slowly while warm

Usage in Traditions: Drink 1 cup after meals for prevention, or at the first sign of indigestion. Can enjoy up to 4 cups daily. For acute indigestion, sip every 15 minutes until relief comes.

Herbal Insights: Peppermint contains menthol, which relaxes the smooth muscles of your digestive tract, allowing trapped gas to pass and reducing spasms. It also stimulates bile flow, helping your body digest fats more efficiently. The aromatic oils have antimicrobial properties that can help rebalance gut flora.

Safety Note: *May worsen heartburn in some people by relaxing the esophageal sphincter. Avoid if you have GERD or gallstones.*

GINGER-LEMON DIGESTIVE TONIC

Chinese sailors chewed ginger root to prevent seasickness over 2,000 years ago. This same root has been starting mornings and settling stomachs across cultures ever since.

What You'll Need:

» 2-inch piece fresh ginger root
» Juice of 1/2 lemon
» 1 tablespoon raw honey
» Pinch of cayenne pepper (optional)
» 1 cup warm water

HOW TO MAKE IT:
1. Peel and grate the ginger root finely
2. Place grated ginger in a mug
3. Add lemon juice and honey
4. Pour warm (not boiling) water over mixture
5. Stir well and let steep 5 minutes
6. Strain if desired, or drink with the bits
7. Add cayenne for extra warming power

USAGE IN TRADITIONS: Drink first thing in the morning on an empty stomach, or 15 minutes before meals. Can also sip throughout the day for ongoing digestive support.

HERBAL INSIGHTS: Ginger contains gingerols and shogaols that stimulate digestive secretions and speed up stomach emptying, preventing that heavy, sluggish feeling. Lemon juice stimulates liver function and bile production, essential for fat digestion. Raw honey provides enzymes and prebiotics that support gut health.

SAFETY NOTE: *May increase acid production—use caution with ulcers. Start with less ginger if you're sensitive to spicy foods.*

CHAMOMILE ANTI-SPASM TEA

Peter Rabbit's mother knew best when she gave him chamomile tea for his stomach ache. This gentle flower has been soothing upset tummies since ancient Egyptian times.

WHAT YOU'LL NEED:
» 3 tablespoons fresh chamomile flowers (or 2 tablespoons dried)
» 1 cup boiling water
» 1 teaspoon honey (optional)

HOW TO MAKE IT:
1. Place chamomile flowers in a tea strainer or pot
2. Pour boiling water over flowers
3. Cover immediately to trap the volatile oils

4. Steep for 10-15 minutes for medicinal strength
5. Strain and press flowers to extract all liquid
6. Add honey if desired

USAGE IN TRADITIONS: Drink 1 cup three times daily between meals for chronic issues, or as needed for acute cramping. Safe for children over 1 year—use half the amount of herbs.

HERBAL INSIGHts: Chamomile contains compounds called azulenes that reduce inflammation and spasms in the digestive tract. Its bitter principles stimulate digestive secretions while its volatile oils calm nervous tension. This makes it perfect for stress-related digestive issues—when your stomach ties itself in knots. It's like a gentle hug for your entire digestive system.

SAFETY NOTE: *Avoid if allergic to ragweed or other plants in the daisy family. May increase the effects of blood-thinning medications.*

FENNEL SEED AFTER-MEAL BLEND

Ever wonder why Indian restaurants offer those colorful seeds after meals? This ancient practice combines fennel, anise, and other seeds to prevent gas and freshen breath—a tradition spanning thousands of years.

WHAT YOU'LL NEED:
» 2 tablespoons fennel seeds
» 1 tablespoon anise seeds
» 1 tablespoon coriander seeds
» 1 teaspoon cardamom seeds
» Small skillet for toasting

HOW TO MAKE IT:
1. Heat skillet over medium-low heat
2. Add all seeds to dry skillet
3. Toast gently for 2-3 minutes until fragrant
4. Stir constantly to prevent burning
5. Remove from heat and let cool
6. Store in an airtight container
7. Can also grind into powder for tea

Usage in Traditions: Chew 1/2 teaspoon of the seed blend after meals, or steep 1 teaspoon in hot water for 10 minutes for tea. Can use up to 3 times daily.

Herbal Insights: Fennel seeds contain volatile oils that relax intestinal spasms and help expel gas—they're nature's Gas-X. The seeds also stimulate digestive enzyme production and have antimicrobial properties that help maintain healthy gut flora. Anise and coriander work similarly, while cardamom adds warmth and helps with nausea. Chewing the seeds also stimulates saliva production, beginning the digestive process right in your mouth.

Safety Note: *Generally very safe. Fennel may have mild estrogenic effects—use moderately during pregnancy.*

SLIPPERY ELM GRUEL FOR ACID REFLUX

Native Americans taught colonists to use slippery elm bark for digestive troubles. During the American Revolution, soldiers survived on slippery elm porridge when food was scarce.

What You'll Need:
» 1 tablespoon slippery elm bark powder
» 1 cup warm water
» 1 teaspoon honey
» Pinch of cinnamon (optional)

How to Make It:
1. Place slippery elm powder in a bowl
2. Add a small amount of cold water to make paste
3. Stir until smooth with no lumps
4. Slowly add warm water while stirring
5. Mix until reaching thin porridge consistency
6. Add honey and cinnamon if desired
7. Drink immediately before it thickens too much

Usage in Traditions: Drink 1/2 cup before meals and before bed. Can take up to 4 times daily. For acute reflux, take at first sign of discomfort.

Herbal Insights: Slippery elm contains mucilage—a gel-like substance that coats and soothes the entire digestive tract from mouth to stomach. This protective barrier shields irritated tissues from stomach acid while they heal. It also stimulates nerve endings in the gastrointestinal tract, increasing mucus secretion which further protects the stomach lining. Think of it as nature's Pepto-Bismol, but better.

SAFETY NOTE: *Take medications 1 hour before or 2 hours after, as the coating may slow absorption.*

DANDELION ROOT BITTER TINCTURE

Medieval physicians called dandelion "piss-en-lit" (wet the bed) for its diuretic properties. But its true gift is stimulating sluggish digestion—those bitter compounds are pure gold.

WHAT YOU'LL NEED:
- 1/2 cup dried dandelion root (or 1 cup fresh)
- 1 cup vodka or apple cider vinegar
- Glass jar with tight lid
- Coffee filter for straining

HOW TO MAKE IT:
1. Chop dandelion root into small pieces
2. Place in glass jar
3. Cover completely with vodka or vinegar
4. Add more liquid if needed—roots should be submerged
5. Cap tightly and label with date
6. Shake daily for 4 weeks
7. Strain through coffee filter, squeeze out all liquid
8. Store in dark glass bottles

USAGE IN TRADITIONS: Take 30 drops (about 1/2 teaspoon) in small amount of water 15 minutes before meals. Can use up to 3 times daily.

HERBAL INSIGHts: Dandelion root is a classic bitter herb—those compounds that make you pucker actually trigger a cascade of digestive secretions. When bitter receptors on your tongue are activated, they signal your stomach to produce acid, your liver to release bile, and your pancreas to secrete enzymes. This prepares your entire system for incoming food.

SAFETY NOTE: *Avoid with gallstones or bile duct obstruction. May increase stomach acid—use caution with ulcers.*

MEADOWSWEET HEARTBURN RELIEF

Meadowsweet gave us aspirin—but unlike its synthetic cousin, the whole plant actually protects the stomach. Medieval brewers added it to mead, hence "meadowsweet."

WHAT YOU'LL NEED:
» 2 tablespoons dried meadowsweet herb
» 1 cup boiling water
» Honey to taste (optional)

HOW TO MAKE IT:
1. Place meadowsweet in teapot or jar
2. Pour boiling water over herb
3. Cover and steep 15 minutes
4. Strain while warm
5. Add honey if desired
6. Drink warm or at room temperature

USAGE IN TRADITIONS: Drink 1 cup after meals or when heartburn strikes. Can take up to 4 cups daily for acute issues, 2 cups daily for maintenance.

HERBAL INSIGHTs: Meadowsweet contains salicylates (aspirin-like compounds) that reduce inflammation, but it also has tannins and mucilage that protect the stomach lining—a beautiful balance. It reduces excess acid production while soothing inflamed tissues. The herb also has mild antimicrobial properties that may help with H. pylori, a bacteria linked to ulcers. Unlike antacids that just neutralize acid, meadowsweet helps normalize acid production. It's particularly good for heartburn with a inflammatory component.

SAFETY NOTE: *Avoid if allergic to aspirin. Not for children with fever due to theoretical Reye's syndrome risk.*

CARAWAY-ANISE GAS RELIEF TEA

Medieval monks grew caraway in their medicinal gardens specifically for digestive troubles. They'd chew the seeds while copying manuscripts to prevent stomach rumbles!

What You'll Need:
- » 1 teaspoon caraway seeds
- » 1 teaspoon anise seeds
- » 1 teaspoon fennel seeds
- » 1 cup boiling water

How to Make It:
1. Lightly crush all seeds with mortar and pestle
2. Place crushed seeds in tea strainer
3. Pour boiling water over seeds
4. Cover and steep 10 minutes
5. Strain out seeds
6. Drink warm

Usage in Traditions: Drink 1 cup after gas-producing meals or at first sign of bloating. Can drink up to 3 cups daily. For infants with colic, give 1-2 teaspoons of weak tea.

Herbal Insights: These three seeds are the traditional European trio for gas relief. They contain volatile oils that relax the smooth muscle of the intestines, allowing trapped gas to pass more easily. They also have antimicrobial properties that help reduce gas-producing bacteria in the gut. The seeds stimulate digestive secretions, helping break down foods that commonly cause gas. This combination is so effective it's been used in gripe water for centuries.

Safety Note: *Start with weak tea for infants and increase strength as needed.*

MARSHMALLOW ROOT INFUSION

Before marshmallows became sugary pillows, they were medicinal lozenges made from this plant's root. Ancient Greeks used it for digestive troubles over 2,000 years ago.

What You'll Need:
- » 1/4 cup dried marshmallow root

» 1 quart cold water
» Glass jar
» Fine mesh strainer

HOW TO MAKE IT:
1. Place marshmallow root in jar
2. Cover with cold water
3. Stir well to wet all root pieces
4. Cover jar and let sit overnight (8-12 hours)
5. Strain out root, squeezing to extract liquid
6. The result should be slightly thick and slippery
7. Refrigerate unused portion

USAGE IN TRADITIONS: Drink 1/2 cup before meals and before bed. Can sip throughout the day for acute issues. Use within 3 days.

HERBAL INSIGHts: Marshmallow root is pure mucilage—when mixed with water, it creates a slippery, soothing gel that coats the entire digestive tract. This protective layer shields inflamed tissues from acid and irritants while they heal. The mucilage also acts as a prebiotic, feeding beneficial gut bacteria. Cold extraction preserves the mucilage better than hot water. This is one of the gentlest, most effective remedies for any inflammatory digestive condition, from heartburn to IBS. It's like applying aloe to a sunburn, but for your insides.

SAFETY NOTE: *Take medications separately as coating may affect absorption.*

LICORICE ROOT ULCER SUPPORT

Ancient Egyptian pharaohs were buried with licorice root to sweeten their journey to the afterlife. Turns out it also sweetly heals stomach ulcers—science proved what ancients knew.

WHAT YOU'LL NEED:
» 1 tablespoon dried licorice root
» 1 cup water
» Small saucepan

HOW TO MAKE IT:
1. Place licorice root in saucepan
2. Add water and bring to gentle simmer
3. Reduce heat and simmer 15 minutes

4. Cover while simmering
5. Strain out root pieces
6. Let cool to drinkable temperature
7. Can refrigerate for up to 3 days

USAGE IN TRADITIONS: Drink 1/2 cup three times daily between meals. Continue for 4-6 weeks for ulcer healing, then reduce to once daily for maintenance.

HERBAL INSIGHts: Licorice root contains compounds that increase the protective mucus coating in your stomach and help it resist acid damage. It also has anti-inflammatory properties that reduce irritation and promote healing of damaged tissues. Studies show it can be as effective as some prescription ulcer medications. The root also helps fight H. pylori bacteria, often implicated in ulcers.

SAFETY NOTE: *Can raise blood pressure with long-term use. Avoid if you have high blood pressure, heart disease, or kidney problems. Not for pregnant women.*

GENTIAN APPETITE STIMULANT

King Gentius of ancient Illyria discovered this root's medicinal properties, giving it his name. It's been awakening sluggish appetites ever since—particularly popular in European digestive bitters.

WHAT YOU'LL NEED:
» 1 teaspoon dried gentian root
» 1 cup hot water
» Honey and lemon (optional)

HOW TO MAKE IT:
1. Place gentian root in cup
2. Pour hot (not boiling) water over root
3. Steep for 5 minutes only—longer makes it too bitter
4. Strain immediately
5. Add tiny amount of honey if needed
6. Sip slowly 20 minutes before meals

USAGE IN TRADITIONS: Take 2-4 ounces before meals to stimulate appetite. Start with small amounts—this is powerfully bitter! Can also use 10-20 drops of tincture in water.

HERBAL INSIGHTS: Gentian is one of the most bitter substances known—and that's exactly why it works. The intense bitter taste triggers a reflex that stimulates every aspect of digestion: saliva production, stomach acid, digestive enzymes, and bile flow. It literally "turns on" a sluggish digestive system. This makes it invaluable for elderly people with poor appetite, those recovering from illness, or anyone with weak digestion. The bitter compounds also have antimicrobial properties and may help regulate blood sugar.

SAFETY NOTE: *Avoid with ulcers, heartburn, or excess stomach acid. Not for pregnant women. The bitter taste is intense—start small.*

MILK THISTLE LIVER SUPPORT TINCTURE

Legend says the white veins in milk thistle leaves came from Virgin Mary's milk dropping on them. Whether divine or not, this plant definitely performs miracles for the liver.

WHAT YOU'LL NEED:
- 1/2 cup milk thistle seeds
- 1 1/2 cups vodka (80-100 proof)
- Coffee grinder
- Glass jar with lid

HOW TO MAKE IT:
1. Grind milk thistle seeds coarsely in coffee grinder
2. Place ground seeds in glass jar immediately
3. Cover with vodka, leaving 2 inches headspace
4. Cap tightly and shake well
5. Store in dark place for 6 weeks
6. Shake daily for first 2 weeks
7. Strain through coffee filter
8. Store in dark glass bottles

USAGE IN TRADITIONS: Take 30-60 drops three times daily in water. For liver support, use for 3 months then take a break. Can resume as needed.

HERBAL INSIGHTS: Milk thistle contains silymarin, one of the most researched herbs for liver health. It protects liver cells from damage, helps regenerate damaged tissue, and increases glutathione (your body's master antioxidant). This makes it invaluable for anyone exposed to toxins, taking medications, or dealing with fatty liver. Studies show milk thistle can help reverse liver damage and improve liver function tests.

SAFETY NOTE: *Very safe. May cause loose stools initially. Can interact with some medications by affecting liver metabolism—consult healthcare provider if on medications.*

ARTICHOKE LEAF DIGESTIVE TEA

Ancient Romans prized artichokes so highly that only nobility could afford them. They knew these thistles aided digestion after their legendary feasts—modern science confirms their wisdom.

WHAT YOU'LL NEED:
- 2 tablespoons dried artichoke leaves
- 1 cup boiling water
- Lemon and honey to taste

HOW TO MAKE IT:
1. Crush artichoke leaves slightly to release compounds
2. Place in teapot or infuser
3. Pour boiling water over leaves
4. Steep covered for 10-15 minutes
5. Strain out leaves
6. Add lemon and honey to offset bitterness

USAGE IN TRADITIONS: Drink 1 cup before heavy meals or 2-3 cups daily for general digestive support. Best taken regularly for cholesterol benefits.

HERBAL INSIGHts: Artichoke leaves contain cynarin, which stimulates bile production—essential for fat digestion and cholesterol metabolism. They also protect liver cells and may help regenerate liver tissue. The leaves have been shown to reduce bloating, nausea, and that too-full feeling after rich meals. Studies indicate regular use can lower cholesterol and improve fat digestion.

SAFETY NOTE: *Avoid if allergic to plants in the daisy family or if you have gallstones. May increase bile flow significantly.*

TURMERIC ANTI-INFLAMMATORY PASTE

In India, turmeric is called "haldi" and considered so sacred it's used in wedding ceremonies. Every grandmother has her own golden milk recipe for digestive troubles.

WHAT YOU'LL NEED:
- 1/4 cup turmeric powder
- 1/2 cup water
- 1/4 teaspoon black pepper
- 1/4 cup coconut oil
- Small saucepan

HOW TO MAKE IT:
1. Mix turmeric and water in saucepan
2. Cook on low heat, stirring constantly
3. Add water as needed to maintain paste consistency
4. Cook 7-10 minutes until thick
5. Add black pepper and stir well
6. Remove from heat and add coconut oil
7. Mix thoroughly and store in glass jar
8. Refrigerate for up to 2 weeks

USAGE IN TRADITIONS: Mix 1/2 teaspoon paste into warm milk, tea, or smoothies. Take 1-2 times daily. Can also add to cooking.

HERBAL INSIGHTS: Turmeric contains curcumin, a powerful anti-inflammatory compound that rivals some pharmaceuticals without the side effects. It reduces gut inflammation and supports liver function. The black pepper increases absorption by 2000%, while the oil helps this fat-soluble compound enter your system. Regular use can reduce inflammatory bowel symptoms, improve digestion, and support overall gut health.

SAFETY NOTE: *May increase bleeding risk—avoid before surgery. Can stimulate gallbladder—avoid with gallstones. May lower blood sugar.*

CINNAMON BLOOD SUGAR BALANCE TEA

Cinnamon was once more valuable than gold. Ancient Chinese emperors sought it for digestive troubles and longevity—turns out they were onto something about blood sugar!

WHAT YOU'LL NEED:
» 1 cinnamon stick (Ceylon preferred)
» 1 cup hot water
» 1 teaspoon raw honey (optional)

HOW TO MAKE IT:
1. Break cinnamon stick into pieces
2. Place in mug or small teapot
3. Pour hot water over cinnamon
4. Cover and steep 15 minutes
5. Strain out cinnamon pieces
6. Add honey if desired after cooling slightly

USAGE IN TRADITIONS: Drink 1 cup with meals, especially carbohydrate-rich ones. Can drink up to 3 cups daily. For best blood sugar effects, take consistently.

HERBAL INSIGHTS: Cinnamon helps your cells respond better to insulin, improving blood sugar control after meals. This prevents the spikes and crashes that leave you tired and craving sweets. It also slows stomach emptying, which moderates blood sugar rise and keeps you full longer. The spice has antimicrobial properties that support healthy gut bacteria balance—important since gut health affects blood sugar regulation. Ceylon cinnamon is preferred as it's lower in coumarin, which can be harmful in large amounts.

SAFETY NOTE: *Ceylon cinnamon preferred for regular use. Cassia cinnamon contains more coumarin, which may harm liver in large amounts. Monitor blood sugar if diabetic.*

CALENDULA TEA

Medieval monks called calendula "Mary's Gold" and grew it in monastery gardens. They used it for everything from plague to digestive troubles—we now know it heals inside and out.

WHAT YOU'LL NEED:
» 2 tablespoons dried calendula petals
» 1 cup boiling water
» Honey to taste (optional)

HOW TO MAKE IT:

1. Place calendula petals in teapot
2. Pour boiling water over petals
3. Cover and steep 15 minutes
4. Strain, pressing petals to extract liquid
5. Add honey if desired
6. Drink warm

USAGE IN TRADITIONS: Drink 3 cups daily between meals for acute issues, or 1-2 cups daily for maintenance. Continue for several weeks for gut healing.

HERBAL INSIGHts: Calendula is famous for healing skin, but it works the same magic on your internal "skin"—the mucous membranes lining your digestive tract. It reduces inflammation, fights harmful bacteria while supporting beneficial ones, and stimulates tissue repair. The bright orange petals contain compounds that improve lymphatic drainage, helping remove inflammatory waste products. It's particularly helpful for leaky gut, ulcers, and inflammatory bowel conditions.

SAFETY NOTE: *Avoid if allergic to plants in the daisy family. May stimulate menstruation.*

PLANTAIN SEED CONSTIPATION RELIEF

Not the banana—the humble yard weed! Europeans called plantain "white man's footprint" because it followed colonization. The seeds (psyllium) have been keeping things moving for centuries.

WHAT YOU'LL NEED:
» 1 tablespoon plantain seeds (or psyllium husks)
» 1 cup water or juice
» Additional glass of water

HOW TO MAKE IT:
1. Place seeds in glass of water or juice
2. Stir quickly and thoroughly
3. Drink immediately before it gels
4. Follow with another full glass of water
5. Can also soak overnight for easier drinking
6. If using powder, start with 1 teaspoon

Usage in Traditions: Take once daily, preferably in the evening. Always follow with plenty of water. Can increase to twice daily if needed. Effects usually occur within 12-24 hours.

Herbal Insights: Plantain seeds are pure soluble fiber that absorbs water and forms a gel-like substance in your intestines. This adds bulk to stool and triggers natural peristalsis (intestinal movement) without harsh stimulation. Unlike stimulant laxatives, plantain seeds don't cause dependency—they simply help your body do what it should naturally. The mucilage also soothes inflamed intestinal walls and feeds beneficial bacteria.

Safety Note: *Always take with adequate water—can cause choking or blockage if taken dry. May interfere with medication absorption—take separately.*

BLACKBERRY LEAF ANTI-DIARRHEAL

Cherokee healers used blackberry root and leaves for "summer complaint"—what we now call diarrhea. Civil War soldiers relied on it when dysentery swept through camps.

What You'll Need:
» 2 tablespoons dried blackberry leaves
» 1 cup boiling water
» Honey (optional)

How to Make It:
1. Place blackberry leaves in teapot
2. Pour boiling water over leaves
3. Cover and steep 10-15 minutes
4. Strain out leaves
5. Add small amount of honey if needed
6. Drink warm or at room temperature

Usage in Traditions: Drink 1/2 cup every 2 hours until diarrhea subsides. Can drink up to 4 cups daily. For children, use half strength and give 1-2 tablespoons every hour.

Herbal Insights: Blackberry leaves contain tannins—astringent compounds that tighten and tone inflamed intestinal tissues. This reduces excessive fluid loss and helps firm up loose stools without stopping bowel movements completely (important for letting your body eliminate what's causing the problem). The leaves also have antimicrobial properties that may help with infectious diarrhea. Unlike harsh anti-diarrheal drugs that stop everything, blackberry works gently to normalize function while soothing inflammation. It's especially good for "summer diarrhea" from food or water issues.

SAFETY NOTE: *Don't use for more than 3 days without addressing underlying cause. See doctor for bloody diarrhea or if accompanied by high fever.*

GINGER HONEY FOR NAUSEA

Chinese sailors sucked on ginger to prevent seasickness 5,000 years ago. Confucius supposedly ate ginger with every meal. This combination with honey makes it taste like candy.

WHAT YOU'LL NEED:
- 1/4 cup fresh ginger root, peeled and sliced thin
- 1 cup raw honey
- Clean glass jar

HOW TO MAKE IT:
1. Fill jar 1/4 full with ginger slices
2. Pour honey over ginger to fill jar
3. Stir to coat all ginger pieces
4. Cap tightly and let infuse 2 weeks
5. Can use immediately but gets stronger over time
6. Leave ginger in honey—it candies beautifully
7. Keeps indefinitely at room temperature

USAGE IN TRADITIONS: Take 1 teaspoon as needed for nausea. Can eat the candied ginger pieces too. For morning sickness, keep by bedside and take before rising.

HERBAL INSIGHts: Ginger contains gingerols and shogaols that specifically target nausea receptors in your digestive system and brain. Studies show it's as effective as some anti-nausea drugs for motion sickness, morning sickness, and chemotherapy nausea. The honey provides quick energy (helpful when you can't eat) and has its own antimicrobial properties. Together, they create a remedy that works fast and tastes good enough that kids will take it.

SAFETY NOTE: *Large amounts of ginger may increase bleeding—use moderately if on blood thinners.*

LEMON BALM NERVOUS STOMACH TEA

Charlemagne ordered lemon balm grown in all monastery gardens for its medicinal virtues. Medieval students drank it before exams to calm nerves and sharpen minds.

What You'll Need:
- 3 tablespoons fresh lemon balm (or 2 tablespoons dried)
- 1 cup boiling water
- Honey to taste

How to Make It:
1. Bruise fresh leaves gently to release oils
2. Place in teapot or mug
3. Pour boiling water over leaves
4. Cover immediately to trap volatile oils
5. Steep 10 minutes
6. Strain and sweeten if desired

USAGE IN TRADITIONS: Drink 1 cup when anxiety triggers stomach upset. Can drink up to 4 cups daily. For chronic nervous stomach, drink regularly between meals.

HERBAL INSIGHTS: Lemon balm is unique—it calms both the nervous system and digestive system simultaneously. Its volatile oils reduce anxiety and nervous tension while also relaxing smooth muscle in the digestive tract. This makes it perfect for "butterflies," nervous diarrhea, or that queasy feeling before important events. The herb also has antiviral properties and may help with stress-related cold sores.

SAFETY NOTE: *Very safe, even for children. May enhance sedative medications. Can interfere with thyroid medications in very large amounts.*

BURDOCK ROOT DETOX DECOCTION

Burdock's clingy burrs inspired Velcro, but herbalists prize the root. Japanese call it "gobo" and eat it regularly—they have some of the world's best digestive health and longevity.

WHAT YOU'LL NEED:
- 2 tablespoons dried burdock root
- 2 cups water
- Small saucepan

HOW TO MAKE IT:
1. Place burdock root in saucepan
2. Add water and bring to boil
3. Reduce heat and simmer 20 minutes
4. Cover while simmering
5. Strain out root pieces
6. Can add honey or combine with tastier herbs
7. Refrigerate unused portion

USAGE IN TRADITIONS: Drink 1 cup twice daily, morning and evening. Best taken for 2-4 weeks as a cleansing course. Can repeat seasonally.

HERBAL INSIGHts: Burdock root is a gentle detoxifier that supports your body's elimination channels—liver, kidneys, lymph, and skin. It contains inulin, a prebiotic fiber that feeds beneficial gut bacteria and helps regulate blood sugar. The root also stimulates bile production and helps the liver process toxins more efficiently. Its mild bitter properties improve overall digestion while its mucilage soothes the gut lining.

SAFETY NOTE: *Start slowly as it can mobilize toxins. Drink plenty of water. May lower blood sugar. Avoid if allergic to daisies.*

CHICORY COFFEE SUBSTITUTE

During the Civil War coffee blockade, Southerners turned to chicory root. New Orleans still prefers their coffee with chicory—turns out this "substitute" has its own benefits.

WHAT YOU'LL NEED:
- 2 tablespoons roasted chicory root

» 1 cup hot water
» French press or coffee maker

How to Make It:
1. If using raw root, roast in oven until dark brown
2. Grind roasted root coarsely
3. Use like coffee grounds in French press
4. Add hot water and steep 5 minutes
5. Press and pour
6. Can mix half-and-half with regular coffee
7. Add milk and sweetener as desired

Usage in Traditions: Drink 1-2 cups daily as coffee substitute or addition. Best in morning or after meals. Can help with coffee reduction.

Herbal Insights: Chicory root contains inulin, a prebiotic fiber that feeds beneficial gut bacteria and helps regulate blood sugar. It stimulates bile production, improving fat digestion and liver function. The roasted root has a bitter, coffee-like flavor but without caffeine's jittery effects. It actually supports liver detoxification rather than stressing it like coffee can. The root also has mild laxative properties, promoting healthy elimination. Plus, it helps reduce coffee dependence without withdrawal headaches.

Safety Note: *May stimulate uterus—avoid during pregnancy. Can cause allergic reactions in those sensitive to ragweed family. Start small to test tolerance.*

PAPAYA LEAF ENZYME TEA

Indigenous peoples wrapped tough meat in papaya leaves to tenderize it. The same enzymes that break down meat proteins help your stomach digest heavy meals.

What You'll Need:
» 2 tablespoons dried papaya leaves
» 1 cup hot (not boiling) water
» Honey and lime (optional)

How to Make It:
1. Crush dried papaya leaves slightly
2. Place in teapot or cup
3. Heat water to 160°F (not boiling)

4. Pour over leaves
5. Steep 10 minutes
6. Strain and add honey and lime if desired
7. Drink warm, not hot

USAGE IN TRADITIONS: Drink 1/2 cup with protein-heavy meals. Can also drink between meals for general digestive support. Most effective when taken regularly.

HERBAL INSIGHTS: Papaya leaves contain papain, a powerful enzyme that breaks down proteins into digestible amino acids. This helps prevent that heavy, sluggish feeling after eating meat or beans. The leaves also have anti-inflammatory properties that soothe digestive tissues and antimicrobial effects that help balance gut flora. Unlike the fruit, the leaves are available year-round and contain concentrated enzymes. They're particularly helpful for people with low stomach acid or enzyme production.

SAFETY NOTE: *May increase bleeding risk—avoid before surgery. Not recommended during pregnancy. Can interact with blood-thinning medications.*

CARDAMOM DIGESTIVE CORDIAL

Bedouins add cardamom to their coffee to neutralize caffeine's harsh effects. Vikings brought it from Constantinople, paying nearly as much as for black pepper.

WHAT YOU'LL NEED:
» 1 tablespoon cardamom pods
» 1 cup water
» 1 tablespoon honey
» 1 teaspoon lemon juice
» Small saucepan

HOW TO MAKE IT:
1. Lightly crush cardamom pods to open
2. Place in saucepan with water
3. Bring to gentle simmer
4. Simmer 10 minutes covered
5. Strain out pods
6. Add honey and lemon while warm
7. Can be served hot or chilled

8. Store refrigerated up to 1 week

Usage in Traditions: Sip 2-3 ounces after meals as digestive. Can also add to coffee or tea. For bad breath, chew a pod after eating.

Herbal Insights: Cardamom is called the "queen of spices" for good reason—it addresses multiple digestive issues elegantly. The essential oils stimulate digestive enzyme production while relaxing intestinal spasms. It's particularly good for gas and bloating from rich foods. Cardamom also freshens breath by killing odor-causing bacteria and increasing saliva flow. The warming quality improves circulation to digestive organs without being too heating. In Ayurveda, it's considered one of the few spices that kindles digestive fire without aggravating it.

Safety Note: *Generally very safe. Large amounts may increase bleeding risk. Can trigger gallstone attacks in susceptible people.*

YELLOW DOCK IRON TONIC

During the Irish potato famine, yellow dock kept many from starvation—it's nutritious as well as medicinal. Appalachian midwives gave it to anemic mothers after childbirth.

What You'll Need:
- 2 tablespoons dried yellow dock root
- 2 cups water
- 1 tablespoon blackstrap molasses
- 1 teaspoon apple cider vinegar

How to Make It:
1. Place yellow dock in saucepan with water
2. Bring to boil, then reduce heat
3. Simmer 20 minutes covered
4. Strain out root
5. Add molasses while warm
6. Stir in apple cider vinegar
7. Store in refrigerator
8. Shake before each use

Usage in Traditions: Take 2 tablespoons twice daily with meals. Best taken for 4-6 weeks, then take a break. Can dilute in water or juice if too strong.

Herbal Insights: Yellow dock is unique—it contains iron and also helps your body absorb and utilize iron better. The root stimulates bile production, improving iron absorption in the small intestine. It also has gentle laxative properties that prevent the constipation common with iron supplements. The bitter compounds improve overall digestive function and liver health. Adding molasses provides additional iron and minerals, while vinegar helps extract and preserve the iron. This is how our ancestors treated anemia without pills—and it still works beautifully.

Safety Note: *Contains oxalates—avoid with kidney stones. Start with small doses as it can cause loose stools. Not for children under 2.*

Respiratory and Immune Support

Take a deep breath. Feel that? Your respiratory system is working its quiet magic, bringing life-giving oxygen to every cell. But when cold season hits or allergies flare, this usually silent system demands attention. The herbs in this chapter have been helping humans breathe easier since we first caught cold—which, let's face it, was probably shortly after we discovered fire and started living in smoky caves together.

Supporting Natural Immunity

Your immune system is like a sophisticated security network, with guards at every entrance and a rapid response team ready for invaders. It's not about having an impenetrable fortress—it's about having smart defenses that know when to act and when to stand down.

The herbs that support immunity don't work like antibiotics, killing everything in sight. Instead, they're more like training coaches for your immune system, helping it respond appropriately to threats. Some herbs, like astragalus, strengthen the guards at the gate. Others, like echinacea, rally the troops when invasion is detected. And some, like elderberry, actively interfere with invaders' ability to replicate.

What's fascinating is how many immune herbs also support respiratory health. This isn't coincidence—your respiratory tract is a major entry point for pathogens, so plants that protect these tissues often boost immunity too.

A healthy immune system isn't just about fighting off colds. It's about maintaining balance—strong enough to protect you, wise enough not to overreact. The remedies in this chapter support both aspects, helping you breathe easy through whatever season brings.

Herbal Support for Respiratory Health

ELDERBERRY IMMUNE SYRUP

Elder trees were considered so magical that people would tip their hats when passing by. In Austria, it was customary to kneel before elder trees and recite prayers for protection from illness.

What You'll Need:
- » 1 cup dried elderberries (or 2 cups fresh)
- » 3 cups water
- » 1 cup raw honey
- » 1 cinnamon stick
- » 1 tablespoon fresh ginger, grated
- » 3 whole cloves

How to Make It:
1. Combine elderberries, water, and spices in saucepan
2. Bring to boil, then reduce to simmer
3. Simmer uncovered for 45 minutes until liquid reduces by half
4. Mash berries with potato masher
5. Strain through fine mesh, pressing out all liquid
6. Let cool to room temperature
7. Stir in honey until well combined
8. Pour into glass bottles and refrigerate

Usage in Traditions: Adults: 1 tablespoon daily for prevention, up to 3 times daily when ill. Children over 1: 1 teaspoon daily for prevention, up to 3 times daily when ill.

Herbal Insights: Elderberries contain compounds that actually prevent viruses from entering your cells—like changing the locks before burglars arrive. Research shows they can shorten flu duration by 3-4 days. The berries are also packed with vitamin C and anthocyanins, powerful antioxidants that support immune function. The added spices aren't just for flavor—ginger warms and stimulates circulation, cinnamon has antimicrobial properties, and cloves add antiviral power.

Safety Note: *Raw elderberries can cause nausea. Some people experience loose stools with large doses.*

ECHINACEA COLD FIGHTER TINCTURE

Plains Indians used echinacea for more ailments than any other plant. They called it "elk root" because they observed sick elk seeking it out—nature's pharmacy in action.

What You'll Need:
» 1/2 cup dried echinacea root
» 1/4 cup dried echinacea leaves and flowers
» 2 cups vodka (80-100 proof)
» Glass jar with tight lid

How to Make It:
1. Place all echinacea parts in glass jar
2. Cover completely with vodka
3. Add more vodka if needed—herbs should be submerged
4. Cap tightly and label with date
5. Shake vigorously
6. Store in dark place for 6 weeks
7. Shake daily for first 2 weeks
8. Strain and bottle in dark glass

Usage in Traditions: At first sign of illness: 1/2 teaspoon every 2 hours. For acute illness: 1/2 teaspoon 4-5 times daily for up to 10 days. Not for daily prevention.

Herbal Insights: Echinacea doesn't kill germs directly—it mobilizes your immune system's rapid response team. It increases white blood cell production and activity, helping your body fight infection more effectively. The root contains alkylamides that tingle on your tongue—that's how you know it's potent. These compounds stimulate immune cell activity throughout your body. Research shows it's most effective when taken at the very first sign of illness, not as prevention.

Safety Note: *Not for autoimmune conditions. Don't use continuously for more than 10 days. Rare allergic reactions in people sensitive to daisies.*

THYME COUGH SYRUP

Medieval knights wore thyme sprigs into battle for courage. Turns out it takes courage to face a hacking cough, and thyme delivers on both counts.

What You'll Need:
» 1/2 cup fresh thyme (or 1/4 cup dried)
» 2 cups water
» 1 cup honey
» Juice of 1 lemon

How to Make It:
1. Place thyme in saucepan with water
2. Bring to gentle simmer
3. Cover and simmer 20 minutes
4. Remove from heat and steep 30 minutes more
5. Strain out herbs, pressing to extract liquid
6. Measure liquid and add equal amount honey
7. Warm gently to dissolve honey
8. Add lemon juice and bottle

Usage in Traditions: Adults: 1-2 teaspoons every 3-4 hours as needed. Children over 1: 1/2 teaspoon every 3-4 hours. Can take straight or add to warm water.

Herbal Insights: Thyme contains thymol and carvacrol, powerful antimicrobial compounds that fight respiratory infections. But here's the magic—it's also an expectorant, helping thin and expel mucus, and an antispasmodic, calming cough reflexes. The honey isn't just for taste; studies show it's as effective as dextromethorphan for coughs. Lemon adds vitamin C and helps cut through mucus. Together, they create a syrup that addresses coughs from multiple angles—fighting infection, loosening phlegm, and soothing irritated tissues. Grandma's cough syrup backed by modern science!

Safety Note: *Not for infants under 1 year due to honey. Large doses may cause stomach upset.*

MULLEIN LUNG TEA

Native Americans introduced mullein to colonists, who called it "Indian tobacco" because they smoked the leaves for lung ailments. The soft leaves were also nature's toilet paper!

WHAT YOU'LL NEED:
» 2 tablespoons dried mullein leaves
» 1 cup boiling water
» Fine mesh strainer or coffee filter
» Honey (optional)

HOW TO MAKE IT:
1. Place mullein leaves in teapot
2. Pour boiling water over leaves
3. Cover and steep 15 minutes
4. Strain carefully through fine mesh
5. Strain again through coffee filter
6. This removes tiny hairs that can irritate throat
7. Add honey if desired

USAGE IN TRADITIONS: Drink 2-3 cups daily for respiratory support. For acute issues, can drink up to 4 cups daily. Best taken warm.

HERBAL INSIGHts: Mullein is like a gentle massage for your lungs. Its mucilage soothes irritated respiratory tissues while saponins help break up congestion. The leaves have anti-inflammatory properties that reduce swelling in bronchial passages, making breathing easier. It's particularly helpful for dry, hacking coughs and that tight feeling in your chest. Mullein also has mild antimicrobial properties and may help with respiratory infections. It's one of the safest, most effective herbs for any lung condition—from asthma to bronchitis to simple coughs.

SAFETY NOTE: *The tiny hairs can irritate if not filtered out. No known contraindications.*

SAGE THROAT GARGLE

The Latin name Salvia means "to save"—medieval monks said "why should a man die whilst sage grows in his garden?" They clearly knew about its throat-healing powers.

WHAT YOU'LL NEED:
- 2 tablespoons fresh sage leaves (or 1 tablespoon dried)
- 1 cup boiling water
- 1/2 teaspoon salt
- 1 teaspoon apple cider vinegar (optional)

HOW TO MAKE IT:
1. Place sage leaves in heat-proof container
2. Pour boiling water over leaves
3. Cover and steep 20 minutes
4. Strain out leaves
5. Add salt and stir until dissolved
6. Add vinegar for extra antimicrobial power
7. Let cool to comfortable temperature

USAGE IN TRADITIONS: Gargle for 30 seconds, 3-4 times daily. Don't swallow—spit out after gargling. Make fresh daily for best results.

HERBAL INSIGHts: Sage is powerfully antimicrobial—it can kill bacteria, viruses, and even fungi on contact. Its astringent tannins tighten swollen throat tissues, reducing pain and inflammation. The volatile oils provide numbing relief while fighting infection. Salt draws out excess fluid from swollen tissues and creates an inhospitable environment for pathogens. It's particularly effective for strep throat, though not a replacement for antibiotics when needed.

SAFETY NOTE: *If drinking, avoid large amounts during pregnancy or while nursing as it can reduce milk supply.*

PINE NEEDLE VITAMIN C TEA

Jacques Cartier's crew survived scurvy in 1536 thanks to indigenous peoples' pine needle tea. This "tree remedy" saved exploration and still supports immunity today.

WHAT YOU'LL NEED:
- 1/4 cup fresh pine needles (Eastern white pine preferred)
- 2 cups water
- Honey and lemon (optional)

HOW TO MAKE IT:
1. Rinse pine needles and chop roughly

2. Place in pot with water
3. Bring to simmer (don't boil hard)
4. Cover and simmer gently 5 minutes
5. Remove from heat
6. Steep covered 20 minutes more
7. Strain and add honey/lemon if desired

USAGE IN TRADITIONS: Drink 1-2 cups daily for immune support. Especially beneficial during cold season or when feeling run down.

HERBAL INSIGHTS: Pine needles contain 4-5 times more vitamin C than oranges, plus vitamin A and antioxidants. But there's more—they contain shikimic acid (yes, the stuff in Tamiflu) and compounds that support respiratory health. The aromatic oils open airways and have antimicrobial properties. The tea brings the forest's supports to your mug—grounding, clearing, and strengthening all at once.

SAFETY NOTE: *Only use true pines (Pinus species). Some evergreens are toxic. Not recommended during pregnancy in large amounts.*

HOREHOUND COUGH DROPS

Horehound candy was the original cough drop—every American pharmacy stocked it until synthetic versions took over. Some old-timers still swear nothing works better.

WHAT YOU'LL NEED:
» 1/2 cup fresh horehound leaves (or 1/4 cup dried)
» 1 cup water
» 2 cups sugar
» 1 tablespoon lemon juice
» Candy thermometer
» Buttered baking sheet

HOW TO MAKE IT:
1. Make strong horehound tea with leaves and water
2. Steep 20 minutes, strain, should have 3/4 cup liquid
3. Combine tea and sugar in heavy saucepan
4. Cook over medium heat, stirring until sugar dissolves
5. Stop stirring, cook to hard crack stage (300°F)
6. Remove from heat, add lemon juice
7. Pour onto buttered sheet in small puddles

8. Let cool completely before storing

USAGE IN TRADITIONS: Suck on 1 drop as needed for cough or sore throat. Can use every 2 hours. Store in airtight container.

HERBAL INSIGHts: Horehound contains marrubiin, a compound that thins mucus and stimulates bronchial secretions, helping clear congestion. It also has expectorant properties that trigger productive coughing to expel phlegm. The bitter compounds may help reduce cough reflex intensity. When made into hard candy, it provides sustained throat contact, maximizing soothing effects. The sugar isn't just for taste—it creates a protective coating on irritated throat tissues. These work better than many commercial cough drops because they actually address the cough, not just numb your throat.

SAFETY NOTE: *Large doses may affect heart rhythm or blood pressure. Not for pregnant women.*

EUCALYPTUS STEAM INHALATION

Australian Aborigines used eucalyptus for everything respiratory. During the 1918 flu pandemic, people wore eucalyptus oil-soaked masks—they had remarkably lower infection rates.

WHAT YOU'LL NEED:
» 5-10 drops eucalyptus essential oil
» Large bowl of steaming water
» Large towel
» Timer

HOW TO MAKE IT:
1. Boil water and pour into large bowl
2. Let cool 1 minute (too hot can burn airways)
3. Add eucalyptus oil to water
4. Position face 12 inches above bowl
5. Cover head and bowl with towel
6. Create tent to trap steam
7. Breathe deeply through nose and mouth

USAGE IN TRADITIONS: Inhale steam for 5-10 minutes. Can repeat 2-3 times daily for congestion. Always keep eyes closed during treatment.

HERBAL INSIGHTS: Eucalyptus oil contains eucalyptol, a compound that kills bacteria, reduces inflammation, and acts as a natural decongestant. The steam carries these volatile oils deep into sinuses and lungs where they thin mucus, open airways, and fight infection. The moist heat alone helps loosen congestion, but eucalyptus supercharges the effect. It's like power-washing your respiratory system—clearing out mucus, killing germs, and reducing inflammation all at once. This simple treatment can break up the most stubborn congestion.

SAFETY NOTE: *Never use for children under 2. Always dilute oils. Too much can irritate airways. Keep eyes closed to prevent irritation.*

ASTRAGALUS IMMUNE BROTH

Chinese tradition calls astragalus "huang qi"—yellow leader—because it leads the body's defensive energy. It's been strengthening immunity for over 2,000 years.

What You'll Need:
» 3-4 astragalus root slices
» 8 cups water
» 1 onion, quartered
» 4 garlic cloves
» 2-inch piece fresh ginger
» 2 carrots, chopped
» Handful of shiitake mushrooms
» Sea salt to taste

How to Make It:
1. Place astragalus and water in large pot
2. Bring to boil, reduce to simmer
3. Add onion, garlic, and ginger
4. Simmer 2 hours partially covered
5. Add carrots and mushrooms last 30 minutes
6. Remove astragalus slices (too tough to eat)
7. Season with sea salt
8. Strain for clear broth or leave chunky

USAGE IN TRADITIONS: Drink 1-2 cups daily during cold season. Can use as base for soups. Especially good for building immunity after illness.

HERBAL INSIGHTS: Astragalus is an adaptogen that strengthens your body's defensive energy over time. It increases production of immune cells, enhances their activity, and helps your body adapt to stress (stress weakens immunity). Unlike echinacea which mobilizes immediate defense, astragalus builds long-term resilience. The additions aren't random—garlic and ginger are antimicrobial, shiitakes boost immunity, and the minerals from vegetables support overall health.

SAFETY NOTE: *Avoid during acute illness—it's for building immunity, not fighting active infections.*

FIRE CIDER TONIC

This recipe was popularized by herbalist Rosemary Gladstar in the 1980s, but the concept of vinegar-based tonics dates back centuries. It's folk remedy with attitude!

WHAT YOU'LL NEED:
» 1/2 cup fresh horseradish root, grated
» 1/2 cup fresh ginger, chopped
» 1/2 cup fresh turmeric, chopped
» 1 onion, chopped
» 10 garlic cloves, crushed
» 2 jalapeño peppers, chopped
» 1 lemon, zested and juiced
» 3 cups raw apple cider vinegar
» 1/4 cup honey

HOW TO MAKE IT:
1. Place all ingredients except honey in quart jar
2. Pour vinegar over to cover by 2 inches
3. Use plastic lid (vinegar corrodes metal)
4. Shake well and label with date
5. Let infuse 4-6 weeks, shaking daily
6. Strain, pressing out all liquid
7. Add honey to taste
8. Bottle in glass containers

Usage in Traditions: Take 1-2 tablespoons daily for prevention. At first sign of illness, take 1 tablespoon every 3-4 hours. Can dilute in water or take straight.

Herbal Insights: Fire cider is like sending the cavalry to defend your body. Every ingredient is antimicrobial and immune-boosting: horseradish opens sinuses and fights bacteria, garlic and onion are nature's antibiotics, ginger warms and stimulates circulation, turmeric reduces inflammation, peppers clear congestion, and vinegar helps extract and preserve all these powerful compounds.

Safety Note: *Very spicy—start with small amounts. May irritate sensitive stomachs. Avoid if you have ulcers or acid reflux.*

OREGANO OIL FLU FIGHTER

Greek shepherds noticed animals eating wild oregano when ill. "Oregano" means "joy of the mountains"—though its property is serious business.

What You'll Need:
» 1/2 cup fresh oregano leaves (or 1/4 cup dried)
» 1 cup olive oil
» Double boiler or slow cooker
» Dark glass bottles

How to Make It:
1. Place oregano in double boiler top
2. Cover with olive oil
3. Heat water to gentle simmer
4. Infuse 2-4 hours, never letting oil bubble
5. Strain through fine mesh
6. For stronger oil, repeat with fresh herbs
7. Store in dark glass bottles
8. Label clearly—this is potent remedy

Usage in Traditions: Internal: Mix 2-3 drops in tablespoon of olive oil, take 2-3 times daily for up to 10 days. External: Dilute heavily before applying to skin.

Herbal Insights: Oregano oil contains carvacrol and thymol, compounds that laboratory studies show can kill bacteria, viruses, fungi, and even parasites. It's one of nature's most powerful antimicrobials—like a natural broad-spectrum antibiotic. The oil also has anti-inflammatory properties and may boost immune function. It's particularly effective for respiratory and sinus infections. The olive oil dilution makes it safer while extracting the medicinal compounds.

Safety Note: *Very potent—never use undiluted. Not for pregnant women or children under 10. Can interact with blood thinners and diabetes medications.*

HYSSOP EXPECTORANT TEA

"Purge me with hyssop, and I shall be clean," says Psalms. This biblical herb has been clearing lungs and purifying spaces since ancient times.

What You'll Need:
- 2 tablespoons fresh hyssop (or 1 tablespoon dried)
- 1 cup boiling water
- Honey to taste
- Lemon (optional)

How to Make It:
1. Place hyssop in teapot or mug
2. Pour boiling water over herbs
3. Cover to preserve volatile oils
4. Steep 10-15 minutes
5. Strain out herbs
6. Add honey and lemon if desired
7. Drink while warm

Usage in Traditions: Drink 2-3 cups daily for productive cough and congestion. Best taken between meals. Can use for up to 2 weeks.

Herbal Insights: Hyssop is a powerful expectorant—it helps thin and expel mucus from lungs and bronchial tubes. The volatile oils have antispasmodic properties that calm coughing fits while still allowing productive coughs. It's also antimicrobial, helping fight respiratory infections. The herb stimulates circulation in lung tissue, bringing healing nutrients and immune cells where needed. It's particularly good for wet, phlegmy coughs.

SAFETY NOTE: *Avoid during pregnancy and with seizure disorders. Contains compounds that may trigger seizures in sensitive individuals.*

COLTSFOOT CHEST RUB

Coltsfoot appears before its leaves, hence "son before father." Roman soldiers carried it for respiratory ailments—even Pliny wrote about smoking the leaves for cough.

What You'll Need:
- 1/2 cup dried coltsfoot leaves
- 1 cup olive oil
- 2 tablespoons beeswax
- 10 drops eucalyptus essential oil
- 5 drops peppermint essential oil

How to Make It:
1. Infuse coltsfoot in olive oil using double boiler
2. Heat gently for 2 hours
3. Strain out herbs completely
4. Return oil to double boiler
5. Add beeswax and stir until melted
6. Remove from heat
7. Add essential oils when slightly cooled
8. Pour into tins immediately

USAGE IN TRADITIONS: Rub on chest and upper back 2-3 times daily for congestion. Can also rub on soles of feet before bed. Safe for children over 2.

HERBAL INSIGHTS: Coltsfoot contains mucilage that soothes respiratory tissues even when applied externally—the compounds absorb through skin. It also has anti-inflammatory properties that reduce chest tightness and ease breathing. The infused oil carries these benefits while the essential oils add decongestant power. Eucalyptus opens airways, while peppermint creates a cooling sensation that tricks your brain into thinking you're breathing easier (and then you actually do!). This traditional remedy is perfect for children or when you can't take things orally.

SAFETY NOTE: *Not for internal use due to pyrrolizidine alkaloids. Avoid on broken skin.*

ELECAMPANE ROOT BRONCHITIS RELIEF

Legend says elecampane sprang from Helen of Troy's tears. Medieval monks candied the root for respiratory ailments—it was their bronchitis remedy of choice.

WHAT YOU'LL NEED:
- 1 tablespoon dried elecampane root
- 1 cup water
- Honey to taste
- Fresh ginger slice (optional)

HOW TO MAKE IT:
1. Place elecampane root in small saucepan
2. Add water and optional ginger
3. Bring to gentle boil
4. Reduce heat and simmer 15 minutes
5. Cover while simmering
6. Strain out root pieces
7. Add honey while warm—needs sweetening!
8. Drink hot

USAGE IN TRADITIONS: Drink 1/2 cup three times daily for acute bronchitis. Can use for up to 2 weeks. Best taken hot between meals.

HERBAL INSIGHts: Elecampane is specifically indicated for deep, wet respiratory conditions. It contains inulin and volatile oils that act as expectorants, helping clear thick mucus from bronchial tubes. The root also has antimicrobial properties, particularly against the bacteria that cause respiratory infections. Its warming nature stimulates circulation in lung tissue, bringing healing resources to infected areas. It's particularly effective for that deep, rattling cough that won't clear.

SAFETY NOTE: *May cause allergic reactions in sensitive individuals. Not for pregnancy. Large doses may cause stomach upset.*

GARLIC-HONEY IMMUNE BOOST

During the plague, grave robbers protected themselves with garlic. Egyptian pyramid builders received garlic rations for strength and disease protection. Still works today!

What You'll Need:
- 1 cup peeled garlic cloves
- 1 1/2 cups raw honey
- Clean glass jar
- Wooden spoon

How to Make It:
1. Lightly crush garlic cloves to release oils
2. Place in clean jar
3. Pour honey over garlic to cover completely
4. Stir to remove air bubbles
5. Cap loosely—may ferment slightly
6. Let infuse at room temperature 4 weeks
7. Can use immediately but improves with age
8. Store at room temperature

Usage in Traditions: Take 1 teaspoon of honey with a few garlic cloves daily for prevention. During illness, take 1 tablespoon 3 times daily.

Herbal Insights: Garlic contains allicin, a compound that's powerfully antimicrobial—it can kill bacteria, viruses, and fungi. When preserved in honey, the allicin remains stable and active. Honey isn't just a preservative; it has its own antimicrobial properties and soothes irritated throats. Together, they create a remedy that fights infection while tasting good enough that kids will take it. The fermentation process may create additional beneficial compounds.

Safety Note: *May increase bleeding—use caution before surgery. Can cause heartburn in sensitive individuals. Not for babies under 1 year.*

ROSEHIP VITAMIN C SYRUP

During WWII Britain, citrus imports stopped. The government organized children to gather rosehips for syrup—it kept the nation healthy through the war years.

WHAT YOU'LL NEED:
» 2 cups fresh rosehips (or 1 cup dried)
» 3 cups water
» 1 cup sugar or honey
» Juice of 1 lemon

HOW TO MAKE IT:
1. Remove stems and blossom ends from rosehips
2. Chop roughly and place in saucepan
3. Add water and bring to boil
4. Simmer 30 minutes, mashing occasionally
5. Strain through fine mesh, then cheesecloth
6. Return liquid to pan
7. Add sugar and lemon juice
8. Simmer until syrupy, about 20 minutes

USAGE IN TRADITIONS: Adults: 1 tablespoon daily for prevention, 2-3 times daily when ill. Children: 1 teaspoon daily for prevention, 2-3 times daily when ill.

HERBAL INSIGHts: Rosehips contain more vitamin C than almost any other fruit—up to 60 times more than oranges! They also provide vitamins A, E, and K, plus antioxidants that support immune function. The vitamin C is particularly bioavailable when extracted into syrup. Unlike synthetic vitamin C, rosehips provide the whole complex with bioflavonoids that enhance absorption and effectiveness. This syrup isn't just about preventing scurvy—it's comprehensive immune support that tastes like fruity sunshine.

SAFETY NOTE: *Very safe. The seeds contain irritating hairs—strain carefully. High vitamin C may cause loose stools in large doses.*

NETTLE ALLERGY RELIEF TEA

"Grasping the nettle" means tackling problems head-on. Ironically, this stinging plant is one of the best remedies for the stinging misery of allergies.

WHAT YOU'LL NEED:
» 1/4 cup dried nettle leaves
» 1 quart boiling water

» Glass jar or teapot
» Honey (optional)

How to Make It:
1. Place nettle leaves in heat-proof container
2. Pour boiling water over leaves
3. Cover tightly
4. Steep 4-8 hours or overnight
5. Strain out leaves
6. Reheat if desired
7. Add honey for taste
8. Drink throughout the day

Usage in Traditions: For allergies: Drink 2-4 cups daily, starting 2 weeks before allergy season. For acute relief: Drink 1 cup every 2-3 hours.

Herbal Insights: Nettle is nature's antihistamine—it actually contains compounds that block histamine receptors and reduce inflammatory response to allergens. The leaves are also incredibly mineral-rich, providing nutrients that support immune balance. Regular use can reduce the severity of seasonal allergies without the drowsiness of pharmaceutical antihistamines. The anti-inflammatory properties help with sinus swelling and irritation. Many people find it works better than over-the-counter options.

Safety Note: *Very safe. May interact with blood thinners and blood pressure medications. Dried or cooked nettles don't sting.*

GOLDENSEAL SINUS RINSE

Cherokee peoples used goldenseal for many ailments, especially infections. It became so popular that it's now endangered in the wild—always buy cultivated!

What You'll Need:
» 1 teaspoon goldenseal root powder
» 1/2 teaspoon sea salt
» 1/4 teaspoon baking soda
» 2 cups warm distilled water
» Neti pot or sinus rinse bottle

How to Make It:
1. Boil distilled water and let cool to body temperature

2. Dissolve salt and baking soda in water
3. Add goldenseal powder
4. Mix thoroughly
5. Strain through coffee filter to remove particles
6. Use immediately in neti pot
7. Make fresh for each use

USAGE IN TRADITIONS: Rinse each nostril with half the solution. Use once or twice daily during active sinus infection. Not for long-term use.

HERBAL INSIGHTS: Goldenseal contains berberine, a compound that's powerfully antimicrobial—it can kill bacteria, viruses, and fungi on contact. When used as a rinse, it directly contacts infected tissues, delivering properties exactly where needed. The salt solution helps thin mucus and reduce swelling, while creating an environment hostile to pathogens. This combination can clear stubborn sinus infections that oral medications can't reach. It's like power-washing your sinuses with natural antibiotics. Many find it more effective than prescription sprays.

SAFETY NOTE: *Not for long-term use. Can dry out nasal passages. Always use distilled water to prevent infections. Not for pregnant women.*

WILD CHERRY BARK COUGH SYRUP

Native Americans introduced colonists to wild cherry bark for coughs. It became so popular that it was an official medicine in the U.S. Pharmacopoeia until 1975.

WHAT YOU'LL NEED:
» 1/2 cup dried wild cherry bark
» 2 cups water
» 1 cup honey
» 1/4 cup brandy (optional)
» 1 tablespoon lemon juice

HOW TO MAKE IT:
1. Place cherry bark in saucepan with water
2. Bring to boil, then reduce heat
3. Simmer gently 15 minutes
4. Remove from heat and steep 1 hour
5. Strain out bark

6. Measure liquid, add equal amount honey
7. Warm gently to dissolve honey
8. Add brandy and lemon juice

USAGE IN TRADITIONS: Adults: 1-2 teaspoons every 3-4 hours as needed. Children over 2: 1/2 teaspoon every 4 hours. Shake before use.

HERBAL INSIGHTS: Wild cherry bark contains compounds that suppress the cough reflex—but unlike codeine cough syrups, it doesn't suppress necessary productive coughs. It's particularly effective for dry, hacking coughs that keep you awake. The bark also has mild sedative properties that promote restful sleep. Anti-inflammatory compounds reduce throat irritation that triggers coughing. The honey coats and soothes while providing its own antimicrobial benefits.

SAFETY NOTE: *Contains compounds similar to cyanide—don't exceed recommended doses. Not for children under 2 or pregnant women.*

ANISE SEED CONGESTION TEA

Roman wedding cakes contained anise seeds for good digestion after feasting. Medieval people chewed them to freshen breath and clear phlegm.

WHAT YOU'LL NEED:
» 2 teaspoons anise seeds
» 1 cup boiling water
» Honey to taste
» Lemon slice (optional)

HOW TO MAKE IT:
1. Lightly crush anise seeds to release oils
2. Place in teapot or mug
3. Pour boiling water over seeds
4. Cover and steep 10 minutes
5. Strain out seeds
6. Add honey and lemon if desired
7. Drink hot

USAGE IN TRADITIONS: Drink 2-3 cups daily for congestion. Best taken hot between meals. Can also inhale steam before drinking.

HERBAL INSIGHts: Anise seeds contain anethole, a compound that thins mucus and helps expel it from respiratory passages. They also have antispasmodic properties that calm coughing while still allowing productive coughs to clear phlegm. The seeds are antimicrobial, helping fight respiratory infections. The warm tea itself helps loosen congestion, while the aromatic oils provide additional decongestant effects. It's gentle enough for children but effective enough for stubborn adult congestion.

SAFETY NOTE: *May have mild estrogenic effects. Avoid therapeutic doses during pregnancy.*

FENUGREEK MUCUS THINNER

Ancient Egyptians used fenugreek for embalming—but the living used it for lung problems. Its name means "Greek hay" though its use predates Greece by millennia.

WHAT YOU'LL NEED:
- 2 tablespoons fenugreek seeds
- 2 cups water
- Honey and lemon to taste
- Small saucepan

HOW TO MAKE IT:
1. Soak fenugreek seeds in water overnight
2. In morning, bring seeds and water to boil
3. Simmer 10 minutes
4. Strain out seeds
5. Add honey and lemon while warm
6. Can also eat the softened seeds
7. Drink warm

USAGE IN TRADITIONS: Drink 1 cup twice daily for thick mucus and congestion. Can increase to 3 times daily for acute issues.

HERBAL INSIGHts: Fenugreek seeds are incredibly high in mucilage—when cooked, they create a slippery substance that thins thick, sticky mucus. This makes it easier to cough up and expel phlegm that's stuck in your lungs. The seeds also have anti-inflammatory properties that reduce respiratory irritation. They're particularly helpful for that thick, glue-like mucus that won't budge. The tea tastes like maple syrup (fenugreek is what gives artificial maple syrup its flavor!), making it one of the more pleasant respiratory remedies.

SAFETY NOTE: *Can lower blood sugar—monitor if diabetic. May stimulate uterine contractions—avoid during pregnancy. Start small—can cause digestive upset.*

LINDEN FLOWER FEVER TEA

European village squares traditionally centered around a linden tree where people gathered. The flowers were everyone's fever remedy.

WHAT YOU'LL NEED:
- 2 tablespoons dried linden flowers
- 1 cup boiling water
- Honey (optional)
- Fresh lemon (optional)

HOW TO MAKE IT:
1. Place linden flowers in teapot
2. Pour boiling water over flowers
3. Cover immediately to trap volatile oils
4. Steep 10-15 minutes
5. Strain out flowers
6. Add honey and lemon if desired
7. Drink hot to promote sweating

USAGE IN TRADITIONS: For fever: Drink 1 cup hot every 2-3 hours. Get under covers to promote sweating. For general use: 1-2 cups daily.

HERBAL INSIGHTS: Linden flowers are a diaphoretic—they promote sweating, which is your body's natural cooling system. But unlike forcing a fever down with medication, linden supports your body's process. The flowers also have mild sedative properties that promote rest (essential for healing) and anti-inflammatory compounds that ease the aches accompanying fever. They're particularly gentle, making them perfect for children's fevers.

SAFETY NOTE: *Supports natural fever process—monitor temperature and seek help for dangerous fevers.*

ONION POULTICE FOR CHEST

During the 1918 flu pandemic, families who ate lots of onions had lower infection rates. Onion poultices on the chest were standard treatment for pneumonia.

WHAT YOU'LL NEED:
- 2 large onions, chopped
- 2 tablespoons olive oil
- Clean cloth or old t-shirt
- Plastic wrap
- Towel

HOW TO MAKE IT:
1. Sauté onions in olive oil until translucent
2. Let cool until comfortable to touch
3. Place warm onions on cloth
4. Fold cloth to create packet
5. Place on chest over lung area
6. Cover with plastic wrap to protect bedding
7. Cover with towel to retain heat
8. Leave on 30 minutes to 2 hours

USAGE IN TRADITIONS: Apply once or twice daily for chest congestion. Can leave on overnight for deep congestion. Safe for children over 2.

HERBAL INSIGHTS: Onions contain sulfur compounds that are antimicrobial and help break up mucus. When applied warm to the chest, these compounds absorb through the skin and volatile oils are inhaled. The warmth increases circulation to lung tissue, helping clear congestion. It sounds like folk nonsense, but it works—many people report dramatic improvement in breathing. The sulfur compounds also have anti-inflammatory effects.

SAFETY NOTE: *May cause skin irritation in sensitive individuals. Test small area first. Strong smell may be overwhelming for some.*

HORSERADISH SINUS CLEAR

Medieval monks grew horseradish in medicinal gardens. They discovered what we now know—it clears sinuses faster than anything else in nature!

WHAT YOU'LL NEED:

» 2 tablespoons freshly grated horseradish root
» 1 tablespoon apple cider vinegar
» 1 teaspoon honey
» Small jar with lid

HOW TO MAKE IT:
1. Grate fresh horseradish root finely
2. Mix immediately with vinegar
3. Add honey and stir well
4. Store in small jar with tight lid
5. Use within 1 week for best potency
6. Keep refrigerated

USAGE IN TRADITIONS: Take 1/2 teaspoon as needed for sinus congestion. Can take up to 3 times daily. Have tissues ready!

HERBAL INSIGHTS: Horseradish contains volatile oils so powerful they can clear sinuses in seconds. These compounds stimulate mucus membranes to drain, providing almost instant relief from congestion. The root is also antimicrobial, helping fight sinus infections. Apple cider vinegar adds additional antimicrobial power and helps preserve the preparation. It's not subtle—this is shock therapy for your sinuses. But when you're desperate for relief, subtlety isn't what you need. One dose can clear sinuses that have been blocked for days.

SAFETY NOTE: *Very intense—start with tiny amounts. Can irritate stomach in large doses. Not for people with ulcers or inflammatory digestive conditions.*

LOBELIA ASTHMA SUPPORT

Also called "Indian tobacco," lobelia was smoked by Native Americans for asthma. Samuel Thomson made it famous in his healing system, calling it his "number one herb."

WHAT YOU'LL NEED:
» 1 teaspoon dried lobelia herb
» 1 cup hot water
» Honey (optional)

HOW TO MAKE IT:
1. Place lobelia in cup
2. Pour hot (not boiling) water over herb

3. Cover and steep 5-10 minutes only
4. Strain carefully
5. Add small amount of honey if needed
6. Sip slowly

USAGE IN TRADITIONS: Take 1-2 tablespoons of tea for breathing difficulty. Can repeat every 30 minutes if needed. Do not exceed 1/2 cup daily.

HERBAL INSIGHts: Lobelia is a powerful bronchodilator—it relaxes the smooth muscles of bronchial passages, opening airways for easier breathing. It also helps expel mucus and reduce spasmodic coughing. The herb works quickly, often providing relief within minutes. It's particularly helpful for asthma and bronchitis with spasmodic coughing. However, it's potent remedy that must be used carefully.

SAFETY NOTE: *Potent herb—can cause nausea and vomiting in large doses. Not for pregnant women or children. Start with very small amounts.*

Skin and External Support

Your skin tells your story—every scar a memory, every wrinkle a smile or worry etched in time. As your body's largest organ and first line of defense, skin works tirelessly to protect, regulate, and communicate. When it needs help, plants offer gentle yet effective support. From battlefield wound care to grandma's garden salve, herbal skin remedies have proven themselves through millennia of use.

Herbal First Aid Basics

Building an herbal first aid kit transforms you from helpless bystander to capable caregiver when minor injuries occur. Unlike the stark white world of conventional first aid, plant-based care brings color, scent, and connection to the healing process. A scraped knee becomes an opportunity to apply purple comfrey salve, a bug bite gets soothed with plantain from the yard, and a minor burn meets cooling aloe and lavender.

The beauty of herbal first aid lies in its accessibility. Many remedies grow in your backyard or sit in your spice cabinet. That "weed" you've been trying to eliminate might be exactly what you need for a bee sting. The dried calendula petals brightening your tea shelf double as wound healers. This isn't about replacing emergency medicine—it's about having natural options for life's inevitable minor injuries.

Skin reflects internal health. While these external remedies provide immediate relief, persistent skin issues often signal deeper imbalances. Sometimes the best skin remedy is a liver-supporting tea or a stress-reducing practice. The herbs in this chapter work both ways—addressing immediate skin needs while supporting overall healing.

Topical Applications

CALENDULA SALVE

Medieval healers called calendula "Mary's Gold" and noticed it turned its flower heads to follow the Virgin Mary's movements. More practically, Civil War nurses used it for wound healing.

WHAT YOU'LL NEED:
- 1 cup dried calendula petals
- 1 1/2 cups olive oil
- 2 ounces beeswax
- 20 drops lavender essential oil (optional)
- Double boiler
- Small tins or jars

HOW TO MAKE IT:
1. Place calendula petals in double boiler
2. Cover with olive oil, ensuring all petals are submerged
3. Heat gently for 2-3 hours, never letting oil bubble
4. Strain through cheesecloth, squeezing out all oil
5. Return infused oil to clean double boiler
6. Add beeswax and stir until completely melted
7. Remove from heat, add essential oil if using
8. Pour immediately into containers

USAGE IN TRADITIONS: Apply to minor cuts, scrapes, rashes, dry skin, or any skin irritation 2-4 times daily. Safe for babies' diaper rash and elderly skin.

HERBAL INSIGHTS: Calendula contains compounds that speed cell regeneration, helping wounds close faster and with less scarring. The flowers have anti-inflammatory properties that reduce redness and swelling, plus antimicrobial actions that prevent infection. Unlike harsh antiseptics that can damage healthy tissue, calendula supports your skin's natural healing process. The oil infusion draws out fat-soluble compounds that water-based preparations miss.

SAFETY NOTE: *Rare allergic reactions in those sensitive to daisy family plants. Always test on small area first.*

COMFREY BRUISE BALM

Comfrey's nickname "knitbone" comes from its legendary ability to speed fracture healing. Medieval bone-setters wouldn't work without it—external use only, always!

What You'll Need:
- 1 cup fresh comfrey leaves (or 1/2 cup dried)
- 1 cup coconut oil
- 1 ounce beeswax
- 10 drops arnica oil (optional)
- 5 drops peppermint oil (optional)

How to Make It:
1. Chop comfrey leaves and pack into jar
2. Cover with coconut oil
3. Let steep 2 weeks, shaking daily (or heat gently 2 hours)
4. Strain out leaves completely
5. Melt beeswax in double boiler
6. Add infused oil and stir well
7. Remove from heat, add essential oils
8. Pour into containers immediately

Usage in Traditions: Apply to bruises, sprains, strains, and sore muscles 3-4 times daily. Excellent for sports injuries. Do not use on open wounds.

Herbal Insights: Known as "knitbone," comfrey has been historically associated with supporting the body's natural healing of bruises, sprains, and other closed injuries. It contains allantoin, a compound thought to promote cell regeneration and tissue repair, while also encouraging healthy circulation. Because it may accelerate surface healing, traditional herbalists caution against applying comfrey to deep wounds. Today, it is commonly used externally in salves or poultices for minor injuries.

Safety Note: *External use only—contains compounds toxic to liver when taken internally. Never use on deep or puncture wounds. Not for pregnant women.*

PLANTAIN DRAWING SALVE

Native Americans called plantain "white man's footprint" because it followed European colonization. Ironically, they taught colonists how to use this "weed" for healing.

WHAT YOU'LL NEED:
- 1 cup fresh plantain leaves
- 1/2 cup olive oil
- 1/2 cup coconut oil
- 1 ounce beeswax
- 1 tablespoon activated charcoal (optional)
- 10 drops tea tree oil (optional)

HOW TO MAKE IT:
1. Wilt plantain leaves for 12 hours to reduce moisture
2. Chop finely and place in double boiler
3. Add oils and heat gently 2 hours
4. Strain through cheesecloth
5. Return oil to double boiler, add beeswax
6. Once melted, stir in charcoal if using
7. Remove from heat, add tea tree oil
8. Pour into small jars

USAGE IN TRADITIONS: Apply thickly to splinters, stings, or infected areas. Cover with bandage. Reapply 2-3 times daily until foreign object emerges or infection clears.

HERBAL INSIGHTS: Plantain has remarkable "drawing" abilities—it literally pulls things out of your skin. The leaves contain aucubin, which has antimicrobial properties, and allantoin (like comfrey) which speeds healing. But plantain's special talent is its ability to draw out venom from stings, pus from infections, and embedded objects like splinters. The mucilage in the leaves creates a pulling action as it dries. Adding activated charcoal enhances this drawing power.

SAFETY NOTE: *The drawing action can initially make infections look worse as they surface—this is normal.*

ST. JOHN'S WORT NERVE OIL

Crusaders brought St. John's Wort back from the Middle East. The red oil it produces was thought to be the blood of St. John the Baptist—it's actually hypericin!

What You'll Need:
» 2 cups fresh St. John's Wort flowers
» 2 cups olive oil
» Glass jar
» Cheesecloth for straining

How to Make It:
1. Harvest flowers on a sunny day when fully open
2. Fill jar with flowers, don't pack too tightly
3. Cover completely with olive oil
4. Place in sunny window for 4-6 weeks
5. Oil will turn deep red—this is the magic
6. Strain through cheesecloth
7. Store in dark bottles
8. Label clearly with date

Usage in Traditions: Massage into areas of nerve pain, sciatica, or neuralgia 2-3 times daily. Also excellent for minor burns and sunburn.

Herbal Insights: St. John's Wort has a special affinity for nerves—it can actually help repair damaged nerve tissue. The flowers contain hypericin and hyperforin, compounds that reduce nerve inflammation and pain. When infused in oil and applied topically, these compounds penetrate to reach aggravated nerves. It's particularly effective for shooting pains, sciatica, and the nerve pain following shingles. The oil also speeds healing of burns and wounds, especially those with nerve involvement.

Safety Note: *Can cause photosensitivity—avoid sun exposure on treated areas. Not for use before sun exposure. May interact with medications if used extensively.*

LAVENDER BURN SPRAY

French chemist Gattefossé discovered lavender's burn-healing properties when he plunged his burned hand into a vat of lavender oil. His rapid healing launched modern aromatherapy.

WHAT YOU'LL NEED:
- 1/2 cup aloe vera gel
- 1/4 cup witch hazel
- 20 drops lavender essential oil
- 5 drops peppermint essential oil
- 1 teaspoon vitamin E oil
- Spray bottle

HOW TO MAKE IT:
1. Pour aloe vera gel into measuring cup
2. Add witch hazel and mix well
3. Add vitamin E oil
4. Add essential oils drop by drop
5. Whisk thoroughly to combine
6. Pour into spray bottle
7. Shake well before each use
8. Label with ingredients and date

USAGE IN TRADITIONS: Spray on minor burns, sunburn, or heat rash as needed. Can apply every 30 minutes for acute burns. Keep refrigerated for extra cooling relief.

HERBAL INSIGHts: Lavender essential oil is one of the few oils gentle enough for neat (undiluted) application, but it's even better in this cooling spray. It contains compounds that speed skin regeneration, reduce pain, and prevent infection—the trifecta for burn care. Aloe provides immediate cooling and healing polysaccharides, while witch hazel reduces inflammation. Peppermint adds extra cooling through menthol.

SAFETY NOTE: *For minor burns only. Seek medical care for severe burns. Test essential oils on small area first.*

TEA TREE ANTIFUNGAL CREAM

Australian Aborigines crushed tea tree leaves into paste for skin infections. WWII soldiers in the Pacific carried tea tree oil in their first aid kits.

What You'll Need:
- 1/2 cup coconut oil
- 2 tablespoons shea butter
- 1 tablespoon beeswax
- 30 drops tea tree essential oil
- 10 drops lavender oil
- 5 drops oregano oil (optional for stubborn fungus)

How to Make It:
1. Melt coconut oil, shea butter, and beeswax in double boiler
2. Stir until completely combined
3. Remove from heat and let cool 5 minutes
4. Add essential oils and mix thoroughly
5. Pour into clean jars
6. Let solidify at room temperature
7. Store in cool, dry place
8. Label with ingredients

Usage in Traditions: Apply to affected areas twice daily after cleaning and drying thoroughly. Continue for 2 weeks after symptoms disappear to prevent recurrence.

Herbal Insights: Tea tree oil contains terpinen-4-ol, a compound that destroys fungal cell walls—literally melting them away. It's effective against athlete's foot, ringworm, nail fungus, and candida. Unlike pharmaceutical antifungals that fungi can develop resistance to, tea tree oil attacks through multiple mechanisms. The coconut oil base isn't random—it contains caprylic acid, another antifungal compound. Together they create an environment where fungus simply can't survive. The cream penetrates deeply while creating a protective barrier.

Safety Note: *Can cause skin irritation in sensitive individuals. Always dilute tea tree oil. Not for internal use. Keep away from pets.*

CHICKWEED ITCH RELIEF

Chickweed's name comes from its popularity with chickens, but humans have used it for itchy skin since ancient times. It often grows where it's needed most!

WHAT YOU'LL NEED:
- 2 cups fresh chickweed
- 1 cup oatmeal
- 2 cups cool water
- Blender
- Cheesecloth or fine strainer

HOW TO MAKE IT:
1. Rinse chickweed and remove any brown bits
2. Place in blender with oatmeal and water
3. Blend until smooth
4. Let sit 20 minutes to extract properties
5. Strain through cheesecloth
6. Press solids to extract all liquid
7. Pour into spray bottle or bowl
8. Use immediately or refrigerate for 2 days

USAGE IN TRADITIONS: Apply liquid to itchy areas with cotton ball or spray directly. Can also soak cloth and apply as compress. Reapply as needed.

HERBAL INSIGHTS: Chickweed is nature's cortisone cream—cooling, soothing, and anti-inflammatory without side effects. It contains saponins that calm irritated skin and reduce the inflammatory response causing itching. The plant's natural cooling property provides immediate relief. Oatmeal adds its own anti-itch compounds called avenanthramides, creating a double-action remedy. Together they address both the sensation of itching and the underlying inflammation.

SAFETY NOTE: *Some people are sensitive—test small area first. Ensure correct identification as some look-alikes exist.*

ARNICA MUSCLE RUB

Swiss mountain guides have chewed arnica leaves for centuries to prevent muscle soreness after climbs. The flower that thrives in harsh mountain conditions helps us thrive too.

WHAT YOU'LL NEED:
- » 1/2 cup dried arnica flowers
- » 1 cup olive oil
- » 2 tablespoons menthol crystals
- » 1 ounce beeswax
- » 20 drops peppermint oil
- » 10 drops camphor oil

HOW TO MAKE IT:
1. Infuse arnica in olive oil using double boiler for 2 hours
2. Strain out flowers completely
3. Return oil to double boiler
4. Add menthol crystals and stir until dissolved
5. Add beeswax and melt completely
6. Remove from heat
7. Add essential oils when slightly cooled
8. Pour into jars before it sets

USAGE IN TRADITIONS: Massage into sore muscles before or after exercise. Apply 2-3 times daily for muscle strain. Wash hands after application.

HERBAL INSIGHts: Arnica contains helenalin, a compound that reduces inflammation and bruising in muscle tissue. It increases circulation to the area, helping flush out lactic acid and bring healing nutrients. The menthol and camphor create a cooling-then-warming sensation that confuses pain signals while the deep penetration addresses actual tissue damage. Peppermint oil adds extra pain relief and that invigorating scent. Athletes swear by it because it actually speeds recovery, not just masks pain.

SAFETY NOTE: *External use only on intact skin. Arnica is toxic internally. Can cause skin irritation with prolonged use. Not for open wounds.*

WITCH HAZEL ASTRINGENT

Native Americans taught Pilgrims to use witch hazel for skin ailments. The name comes from its branches being used as divining rods to find water—appropriate for such a healing liquid!

What You'll Need:
- 1 cup witch hazel bark
- 2 cups distilled water
- 1/2 cup vodka (as preservative)
- 10 drops lavender oil (optional)
- 5 drops tea tree oil (optional)

How to Make It:
1. Place bark in saucepan with water
2. Bring to boil, then simmer 30 minutes
3. Cover and let steep overnight
4. Strain through coffee filter
5. Add vodka as preservative
6. Add essential oils if desired
7. Store in glass bottle
8. Shake before each use

Usage in Traditions: Apply to face with cotton ball after cleansing. Can use morning and night. Also excellent for minor cuts, bug bites, and hemorrhoids.

Herbal Insights: Witch hazel contains tannins that tighten proteins in skin, creating an astringent effect that shrinks pores and reduces oiliness. It's anti-inflammatory, reducing redness and swelling from acne or irritation. The bark also has antimicrobial properties that help prevent breakouts. Unlike harsh commercial astringents, witch hazel maintains skin's moisture balance while removing excess oil. It's like a reset button for your skin—tightening, toning, and clarifying without stripping.

Safety Note: *May cause dryness with overuse. Always use alcohol-free or low-alcohol versions on sensitive skin.*

ROSE HIP SEED OIL SERUM

Chilean women have used rose hip seed oil for centuries to maintain youthful skin in the harsh Andes climate. Science now confirms it's one of nature's best anti-aging treatments.

WHAT YOU'LL NEED:
- 2 tablespoons rose hip seed oil
- 1 tablespoon jojoba oil
- 1 teaspoon vitamin E oil
- 5 drops frankincense essential oil
- 3 drops geranium essential oil
- Dark glass dropper bottle

HOW TO MAKE IT:
1. Pour rose hip seed oil into measuring cup
2. Add jojoba and vitamin E oils
3. Add essential oils drop by drop
4. Mix gently but thoroughly
5. Pour into dropper bottle using funnel
6. Cap tightly and shake gently
7. Label with ingredients and date
8. Store in cool, dark place

USAGE IN TRADITIONS: Apply 3-5 drops to clean face and neck nightly. Pat gently into skin. Can use morning and night for mature skin.

HERBAL INSIGHts: Rose hip seed oil is packed with vitamin A (natural retinol), vitamin C, and essential fatty acids—the trifecta for skin regeneration. It penetrates deeply, stimulating collagen production and cell turnover. The oil reduces hyperpigmentation, softens fine lines, and improves skin texture. Unlike synthetic retinoids, it works gently without irritation. Jojoba mimics skin's natural sebum, ensuring deep penetration. Frankincense has been prized for skin regeneration since ancient Egypt, while geranium balances oil production.

SAFETY NOTE: *May cause breakouts in very oily skin. Always patch test. Use sun protection as vitamin A increases photosensitivity.*

ALOE VERA SUNBURN GEL

Cleopatra credited aloe vera for her beautiful skin. Alexander the Great conquered an island just to secure aloe supplies for treating soldiers' wounds.

What You'll Need:
- 1 cup fresh aloe vera gel (from 3-4 large leaves)
- 2 tablespoons coconut oil (melted)
- 1 tablespoon honey
- 20 drops lavender essential oil
- 1 teaspoon vitamin E oil

How to Make It:
1. Slice aloe leaves lengthwise
2. Scoop out clear gel with spoon
3. Blend gel until smooth and frothy
4. Add melted coconut oil while blending
5. Add honey and vitamin E
6. Add lavender oil last
7. Pour into jar and refrigerate
8. Use within 2 weeks

Usage in Traditions: Apply generously to sunburned skin as needed. Can reapply every hour for severe burns. Keep refrigerated for extra cooling.

Herbal Insights: Aloe vera contains polysaccharides that create a protective barrier while delivering moisture deep into burned skin. It reduces inflammation, speeds cell regeneration, and provides immediate cooling relief. The gel contains compounds that actually help repair UV damage at the cellular level. Adding coconut oil prevents the drying that straight aloe can cause, while honey provides antimicrobial protection and additional healing. Lavender speeds skin repair and reduces pain. This combination addresses every aspect of sunburn—cooling heat, reducing inflammation, preventing infection, and accelerating healing.

Safety Note: *Rare allergic reactions possible. For severe sunburn with blistering, seek medical care.*

CHAMOMILE BABY BALM

German mothers have used chamomile for babies since time immemorial. "Alles zutraut" (capable of anything) they called it—perfect for delicate baby skin.

WHAT YOU'LL NEED:
- 1/2 cup dried chamomile flowers
- 1 cup olive oil
- 2 tablespoons beeswax
- 1 tablespoon shea butter
- 5 drops lavender essential oil (optional)

HOW TO MAKE IT:
1. Infuse chamomile in olive oil for 2 hours using double boiler
2. Strain out flowers, pressing to extract oil
3. Return oil to double boiler
4. Add beeswax and shea butter
5. Stir until completely melted
6. Remove from heat and cool slightly
7. Add lavender oil if using (for babies over 3 months)
8. Pour into containers

USAGE IN TRADITIONS: Apply to diaper area with each change. Safe for cradle cap, minor rashes, and dry patches. Can use from birth.

HERBAL INSIGHTS: Chamomile is gentle enough for newborn skin yet effective enough to handle diaper rash. It contains azulene, which reduces inflammation and promotes healing. The flowers have antimicrobial properties that prevent infection without harsh chemicals. Chamomile also soothes the nervous system through skin absorption—calming fussy babies. The olive oil and shea butter create a protective barrier while moisturizing delicate skin. This simple balm addresses everything from diaper rash to cradle cap to general dryness.

SAFETY NOTE: *Rare allergic reactions in daisy-sensitive individuals. Test on small area first. Use unscented for babies under 3 months.*

JEWELWEED POISON IVY WASH

Jewelweed often grows near poison ivy—nature's antidote placed conveniently nearby. Native Americans rubbed the juice on poison ivy rashes for instant relief.

What You'll Need:
- 4 cups fresh jewelweed stems and leaves
- 4 cups water
- Ice cube trays
- Spray bottle

How to Make It:
1. Chop jewelweed roughly
2. Place in pot with water
3. Bring to boil, then simmer 20 minutes
4. Mash plant material while cooking
5. Strain out solids
6. Pour some into spray bottle for immediate use
7. Freeze remainder in ice cube trays
8. Store frozen cubes in labeled bag

Usage in Traditions: Spray on poison ivy rash immediately after exposure and frequently after. Rub frozen cubes directly on established rashes for relief.

Herbal Insights: Jewelweed contains compounds that neutralize urushiol, the oil in poison ivy that causes the allergic reaction. When applied quickly after exposure, it can actually prevent the rash from developing. For established rashes, it reduces itching and inflammation while speeding healing. The plant's juice has a cooling effect that provides immediate relief. Freezing the preparation makes it even more soothing while preserving it for emergency use. This is one of the few remedies that actually counteracts poison ivy's effects rather than just treating symptoms.

Safety Note: *Ensure correct identification—jewelweed has distinctive orange or yellow flowers and exploding seed pods.*

YARROW WOUND POWDER

Achilles used yarrow to treat soldiers' wounds in the Trojan War—hence its Latin name Achillea. Civil War soldiers carried it as "soldier's woundwort."

WHAT YOU'LL NEED:
- 1 cup dried yarrow leaves and flowers
- Coffee grinder or mortar and pestle
- Fine mesh strainer
- Airtight container

HOW TO MAKE IT:
1. Ensure yarrow is completely dry
2. Grind in coffee grinder until fine powder
3. Sift through fine mesh strainer
4. Regrind larger pieces
5. Store in airtight container
6. Label clearly with date
7. Keep in first aid kit
8. Replace yearly for best potency

USAGE IN TRADITIONS: Sprinkle powder directly on clean wounds to stop bleeding. Apply pressure with clean cloth. For nosebleeds, inhale small amount.

HERBAL INSIGHTS: Yarrow has long been valued in traditional herbal practices for its ability to support wound care. It contains compounds believed to help constrict blood vessels and manage bleeding, while also creating a protective barrier when applied as a powder. Herbalists have also associated yarrow with promoting tissue renewal and soothing swelling, making it a go-to for minor cuts, scrapes, and nosebleeds. Its historical use on battlefields highlights its reputation in aiding the body's natural healing processes.

SAFETY NOTE: *Don't use on deep puncture wounds. May cause allergic reaction in sensitive individuals. Not for pregnant women.*

BEESWAX LIP BALM

Ancient Egyptians used beeswax in cosmetics 4,000 years ago. The same recipes, essentially unchanged, still protect lips today—if it ain't broke, don't fix it!

What You'll Need:

- 2 tablespoons beeswax pellets
- 2 tablespoons coconut oil
- 1 tablespoon shea butter
- 1 teaspoon honey
- 10 drops peppermint essential oil
- Lip balm tubes or small tins

How to Make It:

1. Melt beeswax in double boiler
2. Add coconut oil and shea butter
3. Stir until completely melted
4. Remove from heat
5. Quickly stir in honey
6. Add essential oil
7. Pour immediately into containers
8. Let cool undisturbed until solid

Usage in Traditions: Apply to lips as needed throughout the day. Especially important before going outside in harsh weather.

Herbal Insights: Beeswax creates a protective barrier that locks in moisture without clogging pores—your lips can still breathe. It contains vitamin A, which helps repair damaged lip tissue. Coconut oil penetrates deeply to moisturize, while its lauric acid fights bacteria that can cause cold sores. Shea butter adds vitamins and fatty acids. Honey is humectant (draws moisture) and antimicrobial. Peppermint provides that tingly feeling while increasing blood flow for naturally pinker lips.

Safety Note: *Very safe. Avoid mint oils if sensitive. Some people react to propolis in raw beeswax—use refined if sensitive.*

OATMEAL ECZEMA BATH

Oats have soothed skin since ancient Rome. Even Cleopatra bathed in oat-infused water. Sometimes the simplest remedies remain the best.

What You'll Need:
- » 2 cups whole oats (not instant)
- » 1/2 cup dried calendula petals
- » 1/4 cup dried chamomile flowers
- » Large muslin bag or clean sock
- » Food processor or blender

How to Make It:
1. Grind oats to fine powder in processor
2. Add calendula and chamomile
3. Pulse to mix well
4. Store in airtight container
5. For each bath, place 1 cup mixture in muslin bag
6. Tie securely
7. Can make individual bath bags in advance

Usage in Traditions: Run warm (not hot) bath. Place bag under running water, then let float in tub. Squeeze occasionally. Soak 15-20 minutes. Pat dry gently.

Herbal Insights: Oats contain avenanthramides, compounds that reduce inflammation and itching specifically in skin tissue. They also have saponins that cleanse gently while maintaining skin's protective barrier. The beta-glucans in oats form a protective film on skin that locks in moisture. Calendula speeds healing of eczema lesions while chamomile calms inflammation and irritation. Together they create a bath that cleanses, soothes, protects, and heals.

Safety Note: *Make sure tub isn't too slippery from oils. Some people are sensitive to oats—test first.*

TURMERIC FACE MASK

Indian brides have applied turmeric paste before weddings for centuries—the "haldi ceremony" gives skin a healthy glow. Now science confirms its anti-aging benefits.

WHAT YOU'LL NEED:
- 1 tablespoon turmeric powder
- 2 tablespoons plain yogurt
- 1 teaspoon honey
- 1 teaspoon lemon juice
- Small bowl for mixing

HOW TO MAKE IT:
1. Mix turmeric and yogurt until smooth
2. Add honey and stir well
3. Add lemon juice last
4. Mix to creamy consistency
5. Use immediately
6. Make fresh each time

USAGE IN TRADITIONS: Apply to clean face avoiding eye area. Leave on 10-15 minutes. Rinse with warm water. Use 1-2 times weekly. Follow with moisturizer.

HERBAL INSIGHTS: Turmeric contains curcumin, a powerful anti-inflammatory that calms acne, reduces redness, and evens skin tone. It's also antimicrobial, helping prevent breakouts. The spice increases circulation, giving skin that healthy glow. Yogurt's lactic acid gently exfoliates dead cells while probiotics balance skin's microbiome. Honey moisturizes and heals while lemon brightens dark spots. This combination addresses multiple skin concerns—acne, aging, dullness, and uneven tone.

SAFETY NOTE: *May stain fair skin temporarily. Always patch test. Lemon increases photosensitivity—use at night.*

ROSEMARY HAIR RINSE

Hungarian Queen Elizabeth credited rosemary water for keeping her youthful into her 70s. "Hungary Water" became Europe's first recorded perfume and hair tonic in the 14th century.

WHAT YOU'LL NEED:
- 1/4 cup fresh rosemary sprigs (or 2 tablespoons dried)
- 2 cups water
- 2 tablespoons apple cider vinegar

» 5 drops rosemary essential oil (optional)

HOW TO MAKE IT:
1. Bring water to boil in saucepan
2. Add rosemary and remove from heat
3. Cover and steep 30 minutes
4. Strain out herbs
5. Add apple cider vinegar
6. Add essential oil for extra strength
7. Pour into bottle with applicator tip
8. Use within 1 week

USAGE IN TRADITIONS: After shampooing, pour slowly over scalp and hair. Massage into scalp for 2-3 minutes. Don't rinse out. Use 2-3 times weekly.

HERBAL INSIGHts: Rosemary increases blood circulation to the scalp, delivering nutrients to hair follicles and potentially stimulating growth. It contains rosmarinic acid and caffeic acid, antioxidants that protect against hair damage and premature graying. The herb also has antimicrobial properties that keep scalp healthy and may help with dandruff. Apple cider vinegar removes product buildup and balances scalp pH, creating optimal conditions for healthy hair.

SAFETY NOTE: *Don't use rosemary essential oil if pregnant or have seizure disorders.*

PEPPERMINT FOOT CREAM

Roman soldiers rubbed peppermint on their feet before long marches. No wonder they conquered the known world—their feet didn't hurt!

WHAT YOU'LL NEED:
» 1/2 cup shea butter
» 1/4 cup coconut oil
» 2 tablespoons beeswax
» 30 drops peppermint essential oil
» 10 drops tea tree oil
» 10 drops lavender oil

HOW TO MAKE IT:
1. Melt shea butter, coconut oil, and beeswax in double boiler
2. Stir until completely combined

3. Remove from heat and cool 5 minutes
4. Add all essential oils
5. Whisk vigorously to incorporate
6. Pour into jars while still liquid
7. Let cool completely before capping
8. Store in cool place

Usage in Traditions: Massage into clean, dry feet nightly. Pay special attention to heels and any dry areas. Put on socks after application for overnight treatment.

Herbal Insights: Peppermint's menthol creates an instant cooling sensation that relieves tired, achy feet. But it's not just sensory—menthol actually increases blood flow, helping reduce swelling and fatigue. The oil also has antimicrobial properties that combat foot odor and fungal issues. Tea tree adds extra antifungal power while lavender soothes and heals cracked skin. The rich base of shea butter and coconut oil deeply moisturizes rough foot skin.

Safety Note: *Avoid if sensitive to menthol. Can make shower/tub slippery—be careful. Too much peppermint can cause burning sensation.*

ELDER FLOWER EYE COMPRESS

Medieval ladies used elder flower water to maintain bright, clear eyes. It was said to "remove the heat and inflammation of the eyes"—still true today!

What You'll Need:
» 1/4 cup dried elder flowers
» 1 cup distilled water
» 2 chamomile tea bags (optional)
» Cotton rounds or soft cloth

How to Make It:
1. Bring distilled water to boil
2. Pour over elder flowers
3. Add chamomile tea bags if using
4. Cover and steep 20 minutes
5. Strain through coffee filter
6. Let cool to room temperature
7. Refrigerate in glass container

8. Use within 5 days

USAGE IN TRADITIONS: Soak cotton rounds in cool tea. Lie down and place over closed eyes for 10-15 minutes. Use morning for puffiness, evening for tired eyes.

HERBAL INSIGHTs: Elder flowers contain flavonoids and phenolic acids that reduce inflammation and strengthen delicate blood vessels around eyes. They have mild astringent properties that tighten puffy tissues and reduce fluid retention. The flowers also have anti-inflammatory compounds that calm irritated, red eyes. When applied cold, they constrict blood vessels, further reducing puffiness and dark circles. This gentle treatment works better than caffeinated eye creams because it addresses the root cause—inflammation and poor circulation.

SAFETY NOTE: *Always use clean materials near eyes. If eye problems persist, see healthcare provider.*

BURDOCK ACNE WASH

Japanese prize burdock root as food and medicine. Their clear skin might be connected—they've been using burdock for complexion problems for over 1,000 years.

WHAT YOU'LL NEED:
» 2 tablespoons dried burdock root
» 1 tablespoon dried calendula
» 1 teaspoon dried thyme
» 2 cups water
» 1 tablespoon apple cider vinegar

HOW TO MAKE IT:
1. Combine herbs and water in saucepan
2. Bring to boil, then simmer 20 minutes
3. Cover and let cool completely
4. Strain through fine mesh
5. Add apple cider vinegar
6. Pour into bottle
7. Shake before each use
8. Make fresh weekly

Usage in Traditions: Apply to clean face with cotton ball twice daily. Let dry before applying moisturizer. Can also use as spot treatment.

Herbal Insights: Burdock root contains inulin and mucilage that draw impurities from pores while maintaining moisture balance. The root has antibacterial properties that fight acne-causing bacteria without harsh drying. Calendula heals existing blemishes and prevents scarring, while thyme provides additional antimicrobial power. Apple cider vinegar balances skin pH and acts as a natural toner. This wash doesn't just treat surface symptoms—it addresses the underlying imbalances that cause acne. Clear skin through gentle detoxification.

Safety Note: *May cause purging initially. Discontinue if irritation occurs.*

VIOLET LEAF POULTICE

Medieval physicians prescribed violets for "lumps and bumps." The purple flowers that herald spring also herald healing for swollen lymph nodes and cysts.

What You'll Need:
- 1 cup fresh violet leaves
- 2 tablespoons hot water
- Clean cloth or gauze
- Plastic wrap

How to Make It:
1. Gather fresh violet leaves (flowers work too)
2. Chop or crush leaves roughly
3. Place in bowl and add just enough hot water to wilt
4. Let cool until comfortable to touch
5. Place warm leaves on affected area
6. Cover with cloth
7. Secure with plastic wrap
8. Leave on 30-60 minutes

Usage in Traditions: Apply to swollen lymph nodes, cysts, or fibrocystic breasts daily until swelling reduces. Can leave on overnight for stubborn issues.

HERBAL INSIGHTS: Violet leaves have a special affinity for the lymphatic system—they help move stagnant lymph and reduce swelling in nodes and glands. The leaves contain mucilage that soothes inflamed tissues and saponins that help break up congestion. They're particularly effective for hard, swollen lymph nodes that won't budge. The warmth of the poultice increases circulation to the area, helping the body clear whatever is causing the swelling.

SAFETY NOTE: *If lymph swelling persists or is accompanied by other symptoms, seek medical evaluation.*

CAYENNE WARMING SALVE

Native peoples of the Americas used cayenne for warmth and pain relief long before capsaicin was isolated. They knew heat could paradoxically cool pain.

WHAT YOU'LL NEED:
» 1/4 cup cayenne pepper powder
» 1 cup olive oil
» 2 ounces beeswax
» 20 drops ginger essential oil
» 10 drops cinnamon essential oil
» Gloves for handling

HOW TO MAKE IT:
1. Wear gloves throughout process
2. Infuse cayenne in olive oil using double boiler for 2 hours
3. Strain through fine mesh (outside if possible)
4. Return oil to double boiler
5. Add beeswax and melt completely
6. Remove from heat, add essential oils
7. Pour immediately into tins
8. Label clearly as "warming"—this is hot stuff!

USAGE IN TRADITIONS: Apply small amount to sore muscles or cold extremities. Wash hands immediately. Avoid face and sensitive areas. Test on small area first.

HERBAL INSIGHTS: Cayenne contains capsaicin, which depletes substance P—the neurotransmitter that sends pain signals to your brain.

Initially it creates heat, then numbness, then long-lasting pain relief. It dramatically increases blood flow to applied areas, bringing healing nutrients and removing inflammatory waste products. The warming sensation isn't just pleasant—it's therapeutic, helping relax tight muscles and ease joint stiffness. Ginger and cinnamon add their own warming, anti-inflammatory properties. This salve is perfect for arthritis, poor circulation, and chronic pain.

SAFETY NOTE: *Will burn if applied to sensitive areas. Always wash hands thoroughly. Not for broken skin. Keep away from children and pets.*

LEMON BALM COLD SORE CREAM

Melissa, lemon balm's other name, comes from Greek for "honeybee." Bees love it, but viruses hate it—especially the ones causing cold sores.

WHAT YOU'LL NEED:
- 1/2 cup fresh lemon balm leaves
- 1/2 cup coconut oil
- 2 tablespoons beeswax
- 1 tablespoon honey
- 20 drops lemon balm essential oil
- 10 drops tea tree oil

HOW TO MAKE IT:
1. Infuse lemon balm in coconut oil for 2 hours using double boiler
2. Strain out leaves completely
3. Return oil to double boiler, add beeswax
4. Once melted, remove from heat
5. Stir in honey quickly
6. Add essential oils when slightly cooled
7. Pour into small containers
8. Label with date

USAGE IN TRADITIONS: Apply at first tingle of cold sore. Reapply every 2-3 hours. Continue until completely healed. Can use preventively on vulnerable areas.

HERBAL INSIGHTS: Lemon balm contains rosmarinic acid and other compounds that specifically inhibit herpes simplex virus replication. Studies show it can prevent outbreaks when applied early and speed healing of existing sores. The herb works by preventing the virus from attaching to cells and spreading. Coconut oil contains lauric acid, also antiviral, while honey prevents secondary infection and speeds healing. Tea tree adds extra antimicrobial power. This cream attacks cold sores from multiple angles—stopping viral replication, preventing spread, and speeding healing. It's remarkably effective when used at the first sign of outbreak.

SAFETY NOTE: *Don't share containers to prevent spreading virus. Some people sensitive to tea tree oil.*

THYME ANTISEPTIC SPRAY

Ancient Egyptians used thyme for embalming—if it can preserve mummies, it can handle your minor cuts! Medieval knights wore thyme sprigs for courage and protection.

WHAT YOU'LL NEED:
» 1/4 cup fresh thyme (or 2 tablespoons dried)
» 1 cup distilled water
» 1/4 cup witch hazel
» 1 tablespoon vegetable glycerin
» 15 drops thyme essential oil
» 10 drops lavender essential oil
» Spray bottle

HOW TO MAKE IT:
1. Make strong thyme tea with herbs and boiling water
2. Cover and steep 30 minutes
3. Strain thoroughly through coffee filter
4. Let cool completely
5. Add witch hazel and glycerin
6. Add essential oils
7. Pour into spray bottle
8. Shake well before each use

USAGE IN TRADITIONS: Spray on minor cuts, scrapes, or any area needing disinfection. Can use on surfaces too. Apply 2-3 times daily to wounds.

HERBAL INSIGHTS: Thyme contains thymol, one of nature's most powerful antiseptics—it's used in many commercial mouthwashes. The herb is antibacterial, antiviral, and antifungal, making it a broad-spectrum antimicrobial. Unlike harsh chemical antiseptics that damage healthy tissue, thyme actually promotes healing while fighting infection. Witch hazel adds astringent properties that help clean wounds, while glycerin prevents the spray from drying skin. Lavender enhances healing and adds its own antimicrobial properties.

SAFETY NOTE: *Thyme essential oil can irritate—always dilute. Not for deep wounds.*

Stress, Sleep, and Mental Wellness

In our always-on world, peace of mind has become as precious as gold. Your nervous system, that intricate network connecting thoughts to physical sensations, bears the brunt of modern life's demands. When stress builds and sleep eludes, your whole being suffers. The herbs in this chapter offer what our ancestors knew and what we've forgotten—that plants can gently guide us back to balance, helping quiet the mind's chatter and restore the deep rest our bodies crave.

Herbs for the Nervous System

Think of your nervous system as a finely tuned instrument. When it's in harmony, you feel capable, rested, and resilient. When it's out of tune, every challenge feels insurmountable, sleep becomes elusive, and anxiety colors every moment. Herbal allies for the nervous system work differently than pharmaceutical sedatives—they don't knock you out or numb you. Instead, they help restore your natural rhythms.

Some herbs, called nervines, directly nourish and support nerve tissue. Others, known as adaptogens, help your body adapt to stress more gracefully. Then there are the gentle sedatives that promote natural sleep without morning grogginess. Many herbs fit multiple categories—chamomile calms anxiety while promoting sleep, and ashwagandha builds stress resilience while improving rest quality.

What makes herbal support special is the gentleness. These plants have evolved alongside humans, developing compounds that work with our biology rather than overriding it. They remind your nervous system how to find its own balance, like a gentle hand on your shoulder saying, "Remember how to breathe."

Calming and Restorative Support

PASSIONFLOWER SLEEP TEA

Spanish conquistadors named this vine for Christ's passion, seeing religious symbols in its intricate flowers. Native peoples had long used it for insomnia and anxiety.

WHAT YOU'LL NEED:
- 2 tablespoons dried passionflower herb
- 1 cup boiling water
- Honey to taste (optional)
- Lemon balm or chamomile (optional additions)

HOW TO MAKE IT:
1. Place passionflower in teapot or mug
2. Pour boiling water over herb
3. Cover and steep 15 minutes
4. Strain and add honey if desired
5. Drink warm 30-60 minutes before bed

USAGE IN TRADITIONS: Drink 1 cup nightly for chronic insomnia. For acute anxiety, can drink up to 3 cups throughout the day. Best taken regularly for full effect.

HERBAL INSIGHts: Passionflower specializes in quieting circular thinking—those racing thoughts that keep you awake. It contains chrysin and other flavonoids that bind to the same brain receptors as anti-anxiety medications, but more gently. The herb increases GABA, your brain's main calming neurotransmitter. Unlike pharmaceutical sleep aids, passionflower promotes natural sleep architecture, preserving the deep sleep phases essential for restoration.

SAFETY NOTE: May enhance effects of sedative medications. Not recommended during pregnancy.

VALERIAN ROOT TINCTURE

During WWII London bombings, valerian helped citizens cope with stress and sleep despite air raids. The name comes from Latin "valere"—to be strong and healthy.

WHAT YOU'LL NEED:
» 1/2 cup dried valerian root
» 1 1/2 cups vodka (100 proof preferred)
» Glass jar with tight lid
» Patience (and nose plugs—it stinks!)

HOW TO MAKE IT:
1. Place valerian root in jar
2. Cover with vodka, leaving 2 inches headspace
3. Cap tightly and shake well
4. Store in dark place for 6 weeks
5. Shake daily for first week
6. Strain and bottle in dark glass

USAGE IN TRADITIONS: For sleep: 1/2 to 1 teaspoon 30 minutes before bed. For anxiety: 1/4 teaspoon up to 3 times daily. Start with less—some people are very sensitive.

HERBAL INSIGHTS: Valerian contains valerenic acid and other compounds that enhance GABA activity in your brain—the same mechanism as prescription anxiety medications but without the addiction risk. It's particularly effective for sleep-onset insomnia and muscle tension. The root also contains natural muscle relaxants, making it perfect for tension-related insomnia.

SAFETY NOTE: *Don't combine with prescription sedatives. May cause morning grogginess in some. Not for pregnancy or young children.*

LAVENDER PILLOW SPRAY

Queen Elizabeth I demanded fresh lavender in her bedchambers daily. She was onto something—modern studies confirm lavender improves sleep quality and morning alertness.

WHAT YOU'LL NEED:
» 2 tablespoons dried lavender buds
» 1 cup distilled water
» 2 tablespoons vodka (preservative)
» 20 drops lavender essential oil
» Spray bottle

HOW TO MAKE IT:

1. Make lavender tea with buds and boiling water
2. Cover and steep 30 minutes
3. Strain and cool completely
4. Add vodka and essential oil
5. Pour into spray bottle
6. Shake before each use

USAGE IN TRADITIONS: Spray pillow and sheets lightly before bed. Can also mist bedroom air. Reapply as desired. Safe for children's rooms.

HERBAL INSIGHts: Lavender's linalool and linalyl acetate activate the parasympathetic nervous system—your rest-and-digest mode. Studies show inhaling lavender increases slow-wave sleep, the deepest, most restorative phase. It also reduces cortisol levels and heart rate, preparing your entire body for rest.

SAFETY NOTE: *May cause drowsiness—perfect! Some people find lavender stimulating; discontinue if this occurs.*

SKULLCAP ANXIETY RELIEF

American skullcap got its name from the helmet-shaped flowers. Native Americans used it for women's ceremonies and nervous exhaustion—it's still unmatched for frazzled nerves.

WHAT YOU'LL NEED:
» 1/4 cup dried skullcap leaves
» 1 cup just-boiled water
» Honey or stevia to taste

HOW TO MAKE IT:
1. Place skullcap in teapot
2. Pour water that's cooled 1 minute over herbs
3. Cover and steep 20 minutes
4. Strain and sweeten if desired
5. Drink warm or at room temperature

USAGE IN TRADITIONS: Drink 1-2 cups daily for general anxiety. For acute panic, take 1/4 cup every 15 minutes until calm. Can use long-term.

HERBAL INSIGHts: Skullcap is unique—it calms anxiety while actually rebuilding exhausted nerves. Its flavonoids bind to GABA receptors, promoting calm without sedation. But skullcap also contains minerals and compounds that nourish nerve tissue, making it ideal for anxiety from overwork or burnout. It's like meditation in a cup.

SAFETY NOTE: *Ensure proper identification—other plants share the name. Not recommended during pregnancy.*

ASHWAGANDHA ADAPTOGEN BLEND

Ashwagandha means "smell of horse" in Sanskrit—referring to both its scent and its ability to impart stallion-like strength. It's been Ayurveda's premier adaptogen for 3,000 years.

WHAT YOU'LL NEED:
» 2 tablespoons ashwagandha root powder
» 1 tablespoon tulsi (holy basil)
» 1 cup warm milk (dairy or plant-based)
» 1 teaspoon ghee or coconut oil
» Honey and cinnamon to taste

HOW TO MAKE IT:
1. Warm milk gently (don't boil)
2. Add ashwagandha and tulsi
3. Stir in ghee or oil
4. Simmer 5 minutes
5. Strain, add honey and cinnamon
6. Drink warm

USAGE IN TRADITIONS: Drink nightly for deep restoration. Can also take morning for daytime stress resilience. Use consistently for 6-8 weeks for full benefits.

HERBAL INSIGHts: Ashwagandha doesn't just mask stress—it helps your body handle it better. It normalizes cortisol levels, supports thyroid function, and improves sleep quality. The withanolides in ashwagandha act as adaptogens, helping your body maintain balance despite stressors. Adding tulsi doubles the adaptogenic power while the fat helps absorption.

SAFETY NOTE: *May affect thyroid hormones—monitor if you have thyroid conditions. Can cause drowsiness. Not for pregnancy.*

LEMON BALM MOOD TEA

Medieval scholars called lemon balm the "elixir of life." Students drank it before exams to calm nerves while sharpening minds—the perfect combination.

What You'll Need:
» 3 tablespoons fresh lemon balm (or 2 tablespoons dried)
» 1 cup boiling water
» Honey to taste
» Fresh lemon slice (optional)

How to Make It:
1. Bruise fresh leaves gently
2. Place in teapot
3. Add boiling water
4. Cover immediately to preserve oils
5. Steep 10 minutes
6. Strain and sweeten

Usage in Traditions: Drink 2-3 cups daily for mood support. For acute anxiety or sadness, drink warm every 2 hours. Safe for children—use half strength.

Herbal Insights: Lemon balm is liquid sunshine—it genuinely lifts mood while calming anxiety. It contains rosmarinic acid, which influences GABA receptors, and citral compounds that have mild antidepressant effects. The herb also supports cognitive function, helping clear the mental fog that often accompanies low mood.

Safety Note: *Very safe, even for children. May interact with thyroid medications in very large amounts. Avoid therapeutic doses if hypothyroid.*

CALIFORNIA POPPY SLEEP SYRUP

Native Californians used this golden poppy for children's sleep troubles. Unlike its opium poppy cousin, California poppy is gentle and non-narcotic—nature's lullaby.

What You'll Need:
» 1/2 cup dried California poppy (whole plant)
» 2 cups water
» 1 cup honey

» 1/4 cup brandy (optional preservative)

HOW TO MAKE IT:
1. Simmer herbs in water 20 minutes
2. Cover and steep 2 hours
3. Strain, pressing out liquid
4. Add honey to liquid, warm to dissolve
5. Add brandy if using
6. Bottle and refrigerate

USAGE IN TRADITIONS: Adults: 1-2 tablespoons before bed. Children over 2: 1-2 teaspoons. Can repeat once if needed during night.

HERBAL INSIGHtS: California poppy contains gentle alkaloids that promote relaxation and natural sleep without morning grogginess or dependency. It's particularly helpful for overexcited states—when you're "tired but wired." The herb calms nervous system hyperactivity while supporting natural sleep cycles, making it perfect for both adults and children.

SAFETY NOTE: *Non-narcotic and very safe. Mild sedative effects. Not recommended during pregnancy. No risk of addiction.*

CHAMOMILE BATH SALTS

Ancient Egyptians dedicated chamomile to their sun god Ra and used it in embalming. For the living, it's been the ultimate relaxation herb across all cultures.

WHAT YOU'LL NEED:
» 2 cups Epsom salts
» 1/2 cup dried chamomile flowers
» 1/4 cup baking soda
» 20 drops lavender essential oil
» 10 drops chamomile essential oil

HOW TO MAKE IT:
1. Mix Epsom salts and baking soda
2. Add dried chamomile flowers
3. Add essential oils, mixing thoroughly
4. Store in airtight container
5. Shake before each use

USAGE IN TRADITIONS: Add 1/2 to 1 cup to warm bath. Soak 20-30 minutes. Use before bed for best sleep benefits. Safe for children—use 1/4 cup.

HERBAL INSIGHTS: This isn't just aromatherapy—minerals absorb through skin. Magnesium from Epsom salts relaxes muscles and calms the nervous system. Chamomile's volatile oils absorb transdermally, providing systemic relaxation. The warm water itself activates the parasympathetic nervous system. It's a triple-action calm-down treatment.

SAFETY NOTE: *Hot baths can lower blood pressure—rise slowly. Not for those with certain heart conditions.*

HOPS DREAM PILLOWS

Hop pickers were noted for falling asleep on the job—not from laziness but from the soporific effects of hop flowers. King George III slept on hop pillows for his insomnia.

WHAT YOU'LL NEED:
» 1 cup dried hop flowers
» 1/2 cup dried lavender
» 1/4 cup dried mugwort (optional for vivid dreams)
» Small cotton pillowcase or sachet bags

HOW TO MAKE IT:
1. Mix all dried herbs gently
2. Fill small pillowcase or sachets
3. Don't overstuff—needs to be flat
4. Sew or tie closed securely
5. Place inside regular pillowcase
6. Replace herbs every 6 months

USAGE IN TRADITIONS: Place inside pillowcase near your head. The warmth and movement release sleep-inducing oils throughout the night. For children, use lavender only.

HERBAL INSIGHTS: Hops contain methylbutenol, a compound that becomes more sedating as it ages—why hop pillows improve over the first few weeks. The volatile oils are mildly narcotic, promoting deep sleep. Combined with lavender's calming properties and mugwort's dream-enhancing effects, this creates an all-night aromatherapy treatment.

SAFETY NOTE: *Some people find hops depressing—discontinue if mood drops. Mugwort not for pregnancy.*

KAVA STRESS RELIEF TEA

Pacific islanders have shared kava in ceremonies for 3,000 years. It promotes peaceful discussion and conflict resolution—liquid diplomacy that works on personal stress too.

What You'll Need:
- 2 tablespoons kava root powder
- 1 cup warm water (not boiling)
- 1 teaspoon coconut milk (optional)
- Strainer bag or cheesecloth

How to Make It:
1. Place kava in strainer bag
2. Put bag in bowl with warm water
3. Knead and squeeze bag for 5-10 minutes
4. Water should become cloudy brown
5. Add coconut milk if desired
6. Drink immediately

USAGE IN TRADITIONS: Drink 1/2 cup for social anxiety, 1 full cup for deeper relaxation. Effects felt within 20 minutes. Don't exceed 3 cups daily.

HERBAL INSIGHTs: Kava contains kavalactones that bind to GABA receptors, producing relaxation without mental impairment. Unlike alcohol, kava leaves you clear-headed while profoundly relaxed. It's particularly effective for social anxiety and muscle tension. The traditional preparation method extracts the most beneficial compounds.

SAFETY NOTE: *Don't combine with alcohol or medications. Use only water-based preparations. May cause liver issues with poor quality kava or excessive use.*

MOTHERWORT HEART CALM

The name says it all—motherwort has been mother's helper for centuries. It specifically calms heart palpitations from anxiety, earning its Latin name Leonurus cardiaca.

What You'll Need:
- 2 tablespoons fresh motherwort (or 1 tablespoon dried)
- 1 cup boiling water
- Honey to mask bitterness

How to Make It:
1. Place motherwort in teapot
2. Pour boiling water over herb
3. Cover and steep 15 minutes
4. Strain well
5. Add honey liberally—it's bitter!

Usage in Traditions: Drink 1/2 cup as needed for anxiety with heart palpitations. Can take up to 3 cups daily. Tincture works faster for acute episodes.

Herbal Insights: Motherwort specifically targets anxiety that manifests as heart symptoms—racing pulse, palpitations, or chest tightness. It contains leonurine, which relaxes smooth muscle in blood vessels and the heart. The herb also influences the nervous system's control of heart rhythm, making it invaluable for stress-induced cardiac symptoms.

Safety Note: *Not for pregnancy (uterine stimulant). May increase menstrual flow. Check with doctor if you have heart conditions.*

CATNIP CHILDREN'S CALM TEA

Before catnip became famous for driving cats wild, it was the go-to herb for fussy babies. Ironically, what excites cats calms humans—especially little ones.

What You'll Need:
- 1 tablespoon dried catnip
- 1 cup boiling water
- Honey to taste (for children over 1)

» Chamomile or lemon balm (optional)

HOW TO MAKE IT:
1. Place catnip in teapot
2. Pour boiling water over herb
3. Cover and steep 5-10 minutes
4. Strain carefully
5. Cool to appropriate temperature
6. Sweeten if desired

USAGE IN TRADITIONS: Babies 6-12 months: 1-2 teaspoons. Toddlers: 1/4 cup. Older children: 1/2 cup. Give 30 minutes before bed or during fussy periods.

HERBAL INSIGHTS: Catnip contains nepetalactone, which has mild sedative effects in humans (opposite of cats!). It's particularly effective for digestive upset with restlessness—perfect for colicky babies. The herb gently calms the nervous system while easing gas and stomach discomfort that often disturbs children's sleep.

SAFETY NOTE: *Start with small amounts. Not for pregnancy in therapeutic doses.*

WILD LETTUCE PAIN SLEEP AID

Victorian physicians used wild lettuce as a mild alternative to opium. The bitter white sap, when dried, was sold in pharmacies as "lettuce opium"—legal and non-addictive.

WHAT YOU'LL NEED:
» 2 tablespoons dried wild lettuce leaves
» 1 cup boiling water
» Honey and lemon to taste

HOW TO MAKE IT:
1. Place wild lettuce in teapot
2. Pour boiling water over leaves
3. Cover and steep 15 minutes
4. Strain thoroughly
5. Add honey and lemon—it's quite bitter

USAGE IN TRADITIONS: Drink 1/2 to 1 cup 30 minutes before bed when pain interferes with sleep. Not for daily use—reserve for when needed.

HERBAL INSIGHTS: Wild lettuce contains lactucarium, compounds that have mild sedative and analgesic properties. It's particularly helpful when mild pain keeps you awake—like arthritis or muscle aches. The herb doesn't eliminate pain but reduces it enough to allow natural sleep. It also has direct sleep-promoting effects.

SAFETY NOTE: *Use occasionally, not daily. May cause vivid dreams. Not for pregnancy or children. Large doses cause nausea.*

BLUE VERVAIN TENSION TINCTURE

Ancient Druids considered vervain sacred, using it in prophecy rituals. Maybe they foresaw how much modern humans would need it for stress-induced muscle tension!

WHAT YOU'LL NEED:
» 1/2 cup fresh blue vervain aerial parts
» 1 1/2 cups vodka
» Glass jar with tight lid

HOW TO MAKE IT:
1. Harvest vervain when just beginning to flower
2. Chop and pack into jar
3. Cover with vodka
4. Cap and shake well
5. Steep 4-6 weeks, shaking occasionally
6. Strain and bottle

USAGE IN TRADITIONS: Take 30-60 drops in water for acute neck/shoulder tension. Can take up to 4 times daily. Especially helpful before bed.

HERBAL INSIGHTS: Blue vervain specifically targets tension held in the neck, shoulders, and jaw—classic stress storage sites. It contains verbenalin and other glycosides that relax muscle tension while calming the nervous system. The herb is particularly helpful for type-A personalities who hold stress physically.

SAFETY NOTE: *May stimulate uterus—avoid in pregnancy. Large doses cause nausea. Start with small amounts.*

MIMOSA FLOWER HAPPY TEA

In Traditional Chinese Medicine, mimosa flower is called "collective happiness flower." It's been prescribed for grief and sadness for over 2,000 years—ancient Prozac from a tree.

What You'll Need:
- 2 tablespoons dried mimosa flowers (Albizia julibrissin)
- 1 cup boiling water
- Rose petals or lemon balm (optional)
- Honey to taste

How to Make It:
1. Place mimosa flowers in teapot
2. Add optional herbs if using
3. Pour boiling water over flowers
4. Cover and steep 10 minutes
5. Strain and sweeten

Usage in Traditions: Drink 1-2 cups daily for mild depression or grief. Best taken regularly for several weeks. Can drink as needed for acute sadness.

Herbal Insights: Mimosa flowers contain compounds that influence serotonin and dopamine—your brain's happiness chemicals. The flowers specifically address grief and heartbreak, helping lift the heavy feeling in your chest. In TCM terms, they "calm the spirit and uplift the heart." Modern research confirms antidepressant and anti-anxiety effects.

Safety Note: *Generally safe. May interact with antidepressant medications. Not enough research for pregnancy use.*

RHODIOLA ENERGY TONIC

Vikings used rhodiola before raids for strength and endurance. Siberian villagers still give it to newlyweds to promote fertility and vitality—energy for all of life's battles!

What You'll Need:
- 1 tablespoon rhodiola root powder
- 1 cup warm water

» Lemon juice
» Raw honey

HOW TO MAKE IT:
1. Mix rhodiola powder with warm water
2. Stir thoroughly
3. Add lemon juice and honey
4. Drink immediately—don't let it sit
5. Best taken in morning

USAGE IN TRADITIONS: Drink once daily in morning, preferably before breakfast. Use 5 days on, 2 days off. Take for 6-8 weeks then break.

HERBAL INSIGHts: Rhodiola is an adaptogen that specifically fights fatigue while improving stress resilience. It optimizes serotonin and dopamine levels, improving mood and motivation. Unlike caffeine, it provides sustained energy without crashes. The root also enhances mental performance under stress—perfect for demanding periods.

SAFETY NOTE: *May increase anxiety in some. Not for bipolar disorder. Can interact with antidepressants. Start with low dose.*

HOLY BASIL STRESS TEA

Tulsi (holy basil) is planted around Indian homes and temples for spiritual protection. Science now shows it also protects against the damaging effects of chronic stress.

WHAT YOU'LL NEED:
» 2 tablespoons fresh holy basil leaves (or 1 tablespoon dried)
» 1 cup boiling water
» Ginger and honey (optional)

HOW TO MAKE IT:
1. Bruise fresh leaves gently
2. Place in teapot
3. Add boiling water
4. Cover and steep 5-10 minutes
5. Strain and add ginger/honey if desired

USAGE IN TRADITIONS: Drink 1-2 cups daily for stress resilience. Can drink up to 4 cups during acute stress. Safe for long-term use.

HERBAL INSIGHts: Holy basil is perhaps the perfect adaptogen—it normalizes cortisol, blood sugar, and blood pressure while protecting against stress-induced damage. It contains eugenol and other compounds that support mental clarity while reducing anxiety. Regular use builds resilience to all types of stress—physical, emotional, and environmental.

SAFETY NOTE: *May lower blood sugar—monitor if diabetic. Not recommended during pregnancy.*

MAGNOLIA BARK ANXIETY RELIEF

Traditional Chinese Medicine has used magnolia bark for "stagnant qi" manifesting as anxiety for 2,000 years. Modern research shows it genuinely reduces cortisol levels.

WHAT YOU'LL NEED:
- 1 tablespoon magnolia bark
- 1 cup water
- Small saucepan
- Honey and lemon

HOW TO MAKE IT:
1. Add bark to cold water
2. Bring to gentle simmer
3. Simmer 15 minutes covered
4. Strain out bark
5. Add honey and lemon
6. Drink warm

USAGE IN TRADITIONS: Drink 1/2 cup twice daily for general anxiety. Can increase to 3 times daily during high stress. Best taken between meals.

HERBAL INSIGHts: Magnolia bark contains honokiol and magnolol, compounds that bind to GABA receptors while also lowering cortisol levels. It's particularly effective for anxiety with insomnia and that "wired but tired" feeling. The bark also protects the brain from stress-induced damage, making it neuroprotective as well as calming.

SAFETY NOTE: *May cause drowsiness. Not for pregnancy or nursing. Can interact with sedative medications.*

OAT STRAW NERVE FOOD

"Sowing wild oats" originally meant recovering vitality with oat preparations. Medieval monks grew oats specifically for nervous exhaustion—they knew stressed monks were inefficient monks!

What You'll Need:
» 1/4 cup dried oat straw
» 1 quart boiling water
» Mason jar
» Honey (optional)

How to Make It:
1. Place oat straw in mason jar
2. Pour boiling water to fill
3. Cap and steep 4-8 hours or overnight
4. Strain out herbs
5. Reheat if desired
6. Drink throughout day

Usage in Traditions: Drink 2-4 cups daily for nervous system support. Best used consistently for several weeks. Safe for long-term use.

Herbal Insights: Oat straw is literally food for your nerves—it's rich in B vitamins, calcium, magnesium, and other minerals essential for nervous system function. It doesn't sedate or stimulate but rather nourishes depleted nerves back to health. Perfect for burnout, chronic stress, or recovery from illness. It's like a multivitamin specifically for your nervous system.

SAFETY NOTE: *Extremely safe, even for children and elderly. Gluten-sensitive individuals should avoid. No known drug interactions.*

ROSE PETAL GRIEF TEA

Persian poets wrote that roses bloom from the tears of lovers. The rose has always been associated with the heart—both physical and emotional.

WHAT YOU'LL NEED:
» 2 tablespoons dried rose petals (Rosa damascena preferred)
» 1 tablespoon hawthorn flowers
» 1 cup boiling water
» Raw honey

HOW TO MAKE IT:
1. Mix rose petals and hawthorn
2. Place in teapot
3. Pour boiling water over herbs
4. Cover and steep 10 minutes
5. Strain and add honey
6. Drink slowly, inhaling aroma

USAGE IN TRADITIONS: Drink as needed for grief, heartbreak, or emotional wounds. Can drink 3-4 cups daily during acute grief. Safe for long-term use.

HERBAL INSIGHts: Rose petals contain compounds that specifically address grief and heart-centered emotions. They're cooling and astringent, helping "hold" a heart that feels like it's breaking apart. Combined with hawthorn (a heart tonic), this tea supports both emotional and physical heart health. The aromatherapy component is equally important—rose scent directly impacts the limbic system, where emotions are processed.

SAFETY NOTE: *May have mild laxative effect in large amounts. No known contraindications.*

HAWTHORN HEART SUPPORT

Christ's crown of thorns was supposedly hawthorn. Medieval herbalists used it for "dropsy" (heart failure). It remains one of the most researched cardiac herbs today.

WHAT YOU'LL NEED:
» 2 tablespoons hawthorn berries, leaves, and flowers
» 1 cup boiling water
» Cinnamon stick (optional)
» Honey to taste

HOW TO MAKE IT:

1. Place hawthorn in teapot
2. Add cinnamon if using
3. Pour boiling water over herbs
4. Cover and steep 20 minutes
5. Strain and sweeten
6. Drink warm

USAGE IN TRADITIONS: Drink 1-2 cups daily for heart health and emotional support. Best taken regularly for several months. Safe for long-term use.

HERBAL INSIGHts: Hawthorn works on both physical and emotional heart health. It contains oligomeric procyanidins that strengthen heart muscle, improve circulation, and normalize blood pressure. But hawthorn also addresses the emotional heart—it's indicated for grief, particularly loss of loved ones. This dual action makes it invaluable for stress that manifests as heart symptoms.

SAFETY NOTE: *May potentiate heart medications. Consult healthcare provider if on cardiac drugs. Not for acute heart conditions.*

WOOD BETONY HEADACHE RELIEF

Anglo-Saxons said wood betony would protect against "monstrous nocturnal visions"—perhaps referring to stress headaches and nightmares. It was planted in churchyards for protection.

WHAT YOU'LL NEED:
» 2 tablespoons dried wood betony
» 1 cup boiling water
» Peppermint or lavender (optional)

HOW TO MAKE IT:
1. Place wood betony in teapot
2. Add optional herbs if using
3. Pour boiling water over herbs
4. Cover and steep 15 minutes
5. Strain well

USAGE IN TRADITIONS: Drink at onset of tension headache. Can drink up to 3 cups daily. For chronic headaches, use regularly for several weeks.

HERBAL INSIGHts: Wood betony specifically relieves tension headaches originating from neck and shoulder stress. It improves circulation to the head while relaxing muscle tension. The herb also calms circular thinking that often accompanies tension headaches. It's particularly effective for headaches from mental overwork or eye strain.

SAFETY NOTE: *Generally safe. May lower blood pressure slightly. Not for pregnancy in therapeutic doses.*

JASMINE MOOD LIFT OIL

Cleopatra supposedly seduced Marc Antony in rooms filled with jasmine. In India, it's called "moonlight of the grove"—its scent is strongest at night.

WHAT YOU'LL NEED:
- 1/4 cup fresh jasmine flowers
- 1 cup fractionated coconut oil
- Dark glass bottle
- Small jar for infusing

HOW TO MAKE IT:
1. Place fresh flowers in jar
2. Cover with coconut oil
3. Let infuse 24 hours
4. Strain and repeat with fresh flowers
5. Continue for 3-7 days
6. Final strain and bottle

USAGE IN TRADITIONS: Apply to pulse points for mood elevation. Use as massage oil for emotional release. Inhale deeply from bottle for quick effect.

HERBAL INSIGHts: Jasmine contains benzyl acetate and other compounds that directly influence neurotransmitters associated with pleasure and euphoria. Studies show jasmine scent increases beta waves in the brain—associated with alertness and positive mood. It's one of the few scents proven to be as effective as some antidepressants for mild depression.

SAFETY NOTE: *May be too stimulating for some. Not recommended during pregnancy in therapeutic amounts.*

NUTMEG SLEEP MILK

Medieval Europeans carried nutmeg in special graters, adding it to food and wine. They believed it prevented plague—while that's dubious, it definitely prevents insomnia!

What You'll Need:
- 1 cup warm milk (dairy or plant-based)
- 1/8 teaspoon freshly grated nutmeg
- 1 teaspoon honey
- Pinch of cinnamon

How to Make It:
1. Warm milk gently (don't boil)
2. Grate fresh nutmeg directly into milk
3. Add honey and cinnamon
4. Stir well
5. Drink immediately while warm

Usage in Traditions: Drink 30 minutes before bed. Use only occasionally—not for nightly use. One serving is usually sufficient.

Herbal Insights: Nutmeg contains myristicin and elemicin, compounds with mild sedative properties. In small amounts, it promotes peaceful sleep and vivid dreams. The warm milk provides tryptophan, while the ritual of preparation itself signals bedtime to your brain. This traditional remedy works gently without morning grogginess.

Safety Note: *Use only small amounts—large doses are toxic. Not for pregnancy, children, or those on psychiatric medications. Never exceed 1/4 teaspoon.*

DAMIANA MOOD ENHANCER

Ancient Mayans drank damiana tea for "giddiness and love." Mexican folklore says it was the original ingredient in margaritas—explaining a lot about their mood-lifting effects!

What You'll Need:
- 2 tablespoons dried damiana leaves
- 1 cup boiling water
- Honey and lime
- Cinnamon stick (optional)

How to Make It:
1. Place damiana in teapot
2. Add cinnamon if using
3. Pour boiling water over herbs
4. Cover and steep 10-15 minutes
5. Strain and add honey and lime
6. Drink warm

Usage in Traditions: Drink 1 cup for mood enhancement. Can drink up to 2 cups daily. Effects usually felt within 30-60 minutes.

Herbal Insights: Damiana contains compounds that mildly inhibit aromatase, potentially increasing testosterone in all genders—which can improve mood, confidence, and vitality. It also has mild MAO-inhibiting properties, allowing feel-good neurotransmitters to stick around longer. The overall effect is a gentle euphoria and increased sense of wellbeing without sedation.

Safety Note: *May affect blood sugar. Not for pregnancy or with antidepressants. Can cause mild euphoria.*

Women's and Men's Health

Our bodies tell stories of creation, cycles, and change. From the monthly rhythms of menstruation to the profound transformation of menopause, from the miracle of pregnancy to the gradual shifts of andropause, our reproductive systems profoundly influence overall health. The herbs in this chapter have supported these natural processes for millennia, offering gentle wisdom for life's transitions.

Gender-Specific Herbal Support

While we share more similarities than differences, certain herbs have particular affinities for male or female reproductive systems. These plants don't just address symptoms—they support the intricate hormonal dances that orchestrate our reproductive health. Traditional herbalists understood that reproductive vitality reflects overall vitality, that hormonal balance affects everything from mood to metabolism.

For women, herbs offer support through every life stage: easing menstrual discomfort, supporting fertility, nourishing pregnancy, facilitating birth, encouraging lactation, and smoothing the menopausal transition.

For men, herbs support prostate health, hormonal balance, fertility, and vitality. While men's reproductive health has received less traditional attention, many cultures developed sophisticated herbal protocols for male wellness, recognizing that men too experience hormonal shifts and benefit from plant support.

Remember that reproductive health is whole-person health. Stress, nutrition, sleep, and emotional wellbeing all influence hormonal balance. The herbs here work best as part of a holistic approach that honors the wisdom of your body.

Reproductive and Hormonal Health

RED RASPBERRY LEAF PREGNANCY TEA

Native American women drank raspberry leaf tea throughout pregnancy for easier births. Midwives have passed this wisdom through generations—it remains a cornerstone of herbal pregnancy care.

What You'll Need:
» 1/4 cup dried red raspberry leaves
» 1 quart boiling water
» Honey to taste
» Mint or nettle (optional)

How to Make It:
1. Place raspberry leaves in quart jar
2. Pour boiling water to fill
3. Cover and steep 20-30 minutes
4. Strain leaves
5. Add honey if desired
6. Drink warm or cold

Usage in Traditions: First trimester: 1 cup daily. Second trimester: 2 cups daily. Third trimester: 3-4 cups daily. Can drink hot or iced.

Herbal Insights: Red raspberry leaves contain fragarine, a compound that tones uterine muscles, potentially making contractions more efficient. The leaves are also rich in vitamins and minerals essential for pregnancy—iron, calcium, and B vitamins. Regular use may reduce morning sickness, prevent miscarriage, and ease labor.

Safety Note: *Some suggest avoiding in first trimester with history of miscarriage. Always consult your healthcare provider.*

CRAMP BARK MENSTRUAL RELIEF

Native Americans called it "squaw bush" for its effectiveness with women's complaints. The name "cramp bark" says it all—this is nature's muscle relaxant.

What You'll Need:
» 2 tablespoons dried cramp bark

» 1 cup water
» Ginger and cinnamon (optional)
» Honey to taste

HOW TO MAKE IT:
1. Simmer cramp bark in water 15 minutes
2. Add ginger and cinnamon if using
3. Cover and steep 10 more minutes
4. Strain and sweeten
5. Drink hot

USAGE IN TRADITIONS: Start 2 days before period for prevention. During cramps: 1/2 cup every 30 minutes until relief. Can take up to 4 cups daily.

HERBAL INSIGHts: Cramp bark contains scopoletin and viopudial, natural muscle relaxants that specifically target smooth muscle like the uterus. It reduces both the intensity and frequency of cramps without interfering with normal menstruation. The bark also has mild sedative properties, helping with menstrual irritability.

SAFETY NOTE: *Contains natural aspirin-like compounds—avoid if allergic to aspirin. Not for pregnancy.*

DONG QUAI WOMEN'S TONIC

Chinese women have used dong quai for over 2,000 years, calling it "female ginseng." It's said that monks gave it this name after noticing village women who used it maintained youthful vitality.

WHAT YOU'LL NEED:
» 1 tablespoon dong quai root slices
» 1 cup water
» Goji berries and licorice (optional)

HOW TO MAKE IT:
1. Simmer dong quai in water 20 minutes
2. Add goji berries last 5 minutes
3. Strain out herbs
4. Can add licorice for sweetness
5. Drink warm

Usage in Traditions: Drink 1 cup daily, except during menstruation. Best taken for 3 months to see full effects. Can take breaks during period.

Herbal Insights: Dong quai doesn't contain hormones but rather helps your body balance its own hormone production. It improves circulation to reproductive organs, regulates menstrual cycles, and may reduce menopausal symptoms. The root also builds blood, addressing the fatigue common with heavy periods.

Safety Note: *Not during pregnancy, heavy bleeding, or with blood thinners. May increase menstrual flow. Can cause photosensitivity.*

VITEX BERRY HORMONE BALANCE

Medieval monks chewed vitex berries to reduce libido—hence "chaste tree." Ironically, it actually balances hormones rather than suppressing them, potentially improving fertility!

What You'll Need:
» 1 teaspoon dried vitex berries
» 1 cup boiling water
» Honey and lemon

How to Make It:
1. Crush vitex berries slightly
2. Place in cup or teapot
3. Pour boiling water over berries
4. Cover and steep 15 minutes
5. Strain and add honey/lemon

Usage in Traditions: Drink 1 cup each morning before breakfast. Use consistently for 3-6 months. Take 5 days off during menstruation.

Herbal Insights: Vitex works on the pituitary gland, helping regulate the hormones that control your menstrual cycle. It's particularly effective for PMS, irregular periods, and hormonal acne. Rather than adding hormones, it helps your body find its own balance, making it safe for long-term use.

Safety Note: *Not for pregnancy, nursing, or with hormonal birth control. May interact with fertility drugs. Can affect menstrual flow initially.*

BLACK COHOSH MENOPAUSE SUPPORT

Native Americans called it "squaw root" and used it for all female complaints. It became so popular that 19th century patent medicines nearly always contained it.

WHAT YOU'LL NEED:
» 1 teaspoon dried black cohosh root
» 1 cup water
» Peppermint and sage (optional)

HOW TO MAKE IT:
1. Simmer black cohosh in water 15 minutes
2. Remove from heat
3. Add peppermint and sage if using
4. Cover and steep 10 minutes
5. Strain well

USAGE IN TRADITIONS: Drink 1/2 cup twice daily for menopausal symptoms. Can increase to 3 times daily for severe hot flashes.

HERBAL INSIGHts: Black cohosh contains triterpene glycosides that help modulate estrogen receptors without being truly estrogenic. It's particularly effective for hot flashes, night sweats, and mood swings. Studies show it can be as effective as hormone replacement for some women, without the risks.

SAFETY NOTE: *Not for pregnancy or with liver disease. May cause stomach upset initially. Don't use for more than 6 months continuously.*

NETTLE IRON-RICH TEA

European women traditionally ate nettle soup after childbirth to rebuild blood. The sting that makes harvesting challenging disappears with drying or cooking.

WHAT YOU'LL NEED:
» 1/4 cup dried nettle leaves
» 1 quart boiling water
» Lemon juice
» Honey or molasses

HOW TO MAKE IT:

1. Place nettles in quart jar
2. Fill with boiling water
3. Cover and steep 4-8 hours
4. Strain and squeeze leaves
5. Add lemon juice
6. Sweeten with honey or molasses

USAGE IN TRADITIONS: Drink 2-4 cups daily for iron deficiency. Best absorbed on empty stomach with vitamin C. Can drink throughout pregnancy.

HERBAL INSIGHTS: Nettle is incredibly mineral-rich, containing easily absorbed iron along with vitamin C for absorption. It also provides calcium, magnesium, and trace minerals. Unlike iron supplements, nettle doesn't cause constipation and actually improves overall nutrition. It's particularly valuable for women with heavy periods.

SAFETY NOTE: *May affect blood sugar and blood pressure. Fresh plant stings—handle with gloves.*

LADY'S MANTLE HEAVY FLOW TEA

Alchemists collected dew from lady's mantle leaves, believing it could create the philosopher's stone. While it can't turn lead to gold, it can transform heavy periods!

WHAT YOU'LL NEED:
» 2 tablespoons dried lady's mantle
» 1 cup boiling water
» Shepherd's purse (optional for extra strength)

HOW TO MAKE IT:
1. Place herbs in teapot
2. Pour boiling water over
3. Cover and steep 15 minutes
4. Strain well
5. Drink warm

USAGE IN TRADITIONS: Start 3 days before period: 3 cups daily. During heavy flow: 1 cup every 3-4 hours. Can combine with shepherd's purse for severe bleeding.

HERBAL INSIGHts: Lady's mantle contains tannins that have astringent properties, helping reduce excessive menstrual flow. It tones the uterus and helps regulate periods without stopping healthy flow. The herb also contains salicylic acid, providing mild pain relief for cramps.

SAFETY NOTE: *The astringent nature may cause constipation in some. Not for pregnancy.*

SHEPHERD'S PURSE BLEEDING CONTROL

WWI soldiers carried shepherd's purse to stop battlefield bleeding. This humble weed has saved countless lives through its powerful hemostatic properties.

WHAT YOU'LL NEED:
- » 3 tablespoons fresh shepherd's purse (or 2 tablespoons dried)
- » 1 cup boiling water
- » Clean cloth for compress

HOW TO MAKE IT:
1. Pour boiling water over herb
2. Cover and steep 10 minutes
3. Strain, reserving liquid
4. Drink tea immediately
5. Use warm herbs as compress
6. Repeat as needed

USAGE IN TRADITIONS: For heavy menstrual bleeding: 1/2 cup every hour until flow normalizes. For nosebleeds: soak cloth in tea and apply. Seek medical care for severe bleeding.

HERBAL INSIGHts: Shepherd's purse contains peptides that constrict blood vessels and promote clotting. It works quickly—often within 15-30 minutes—to reduce excessive bleeding. The herb specifically targets uterine bleeding without affecting normal clotting elsewhere in the body.

SAFETY NOTE: *Powerful herb—use only for acute bleeding. Not for regular use or during pregnancy. Seek medical attention for severe bleeding.*

FENNEL NURSING TEA

Greek mothers have drunk fennel tea while nursing for thousands of years. Hippocrates himself recommended it for increasing milk supply—ancient wisdom still valid today.

What You'll Need:
» 2 tablespoons fennel seeds
» 1 tablespoon fenugreek seeds
» 1 tablespoon blessed thistle (optional)
» 2 cups boiling water

How to Make It:
1. Lightly crush all seeds
2. Place in teapot
3. Pour boiling water over
4. Cover and steep 10-15 minutes
5. Strain seeds
6. Drink warm

Usage in Traditions: Drink 3-4 cups daily while nursing. Best results when started within first week postpartum. Can drink cold or hot.

Herbal Insights: Fennel contains phytoestrogens that stimulate milk production. The volatile oils also pass into breast milk, helping baby with gas and colic—double benefit! Combined with fenugreek (another galactagogue), this traditional blend can significantly increase milk supply within 24-72 hours.

Safety Note: *May cause gas initially. Not for pregnancy in therapeutic doses. Allergic reactions rare but possible.*

SAW PALMETTO PROSTATE SUPPORT

Native Americans ate saw palmetto berries for food and medicine. Early colonists noticed indigenous men maintained urinary health into old age—the berries were their secret.

What You'll Need:
» 1 tablespoon dried saw palmetto berries
» 1 cup water
» Honey to taste

HOW TO MAKE IT:
1. Simmer berries in water 20 minutes
2. Cover and let cool
3. Strain out berries
4. Add honey if desired
5. Drink warm or cold

USAGE IN TRADITIONS: Drink 1 cup twice daily for prostate health. Best taken with meals. Use consistently for 3 months to see effects.

HERBAL INSIGHts: Saw palmetto contains fatty acids and phytosterols that help prevent testosterone from converting to DHT, the hormone that enlarges the prostate. It specifically reduces nighttime urination and improves urinary flow without affecting hormone levels elsewhere. Studies show it's as effective as some prescription medications.

SAFETY NOTE: *May interact with hormone medications. Can cause mild stomach upset initially.*

TRIBULUS MEN'S VITALITY

Bulgarian Olympic athletes credited tribulus for their success in the 1980s. This spiny plant has been used in Ayurveda and Chinese medicine for male vitality for centuries.

WHAT YOU'LL NEED:
» 1 tablespoon tribulus fruit powder
» 1 cup warm water
» Raw honey
» Pinch of black pepper

HOW TO MAKE IT:
1. Mix tribulus powder in warm water
2. Add honey and black pepper
3. Stir thoroughly
4. Drink immediately
5. Don't let it sit—bitter compounds settle

USAGE IN TRADITIONS: Drink once daily in morning. Take for 8 weeks, then take 2 weeks off. Can repeat cycles.

HERBAL INSIGHts: Tribulus contains protodioscin, which may support the body's natural testosterone production. It doesn't add hormones but rather helps optimize your body's own production. Users report improved energy, muscle mass, and libido. The herb also supports cardiovascular health—important for male vitality.

SAFETY NOTE: *May affect blood sugar and blood pressure. Not for prostate issues. Can interact with heart and diabetes medications.*

GINSENG ENERGY TONIC

Chinese emperors monopolized wild ginseng, believing it conferred immortality. Wars were fought over ginseng territory. Today it's still one of the most valued herbs worldwide.

WHAT YOU'LL NEED:
» 1 tablespoon ginseng root slices (Asian or American)
» 1 cup hot water
» Honey and lemon
» Goji berries (optional)

HOW TO MAKE IT:
1. Place ginseng in cup
2. Pour hot (not boiling) water over
3. Cover and steep 20 minutes
4. Add goji berries last 5 minutes
5. Strain and add honey/lemon
6. Chew the softened root pieces

USAGE IN TRADITIONS: Drink 1 cup in morning for 3 weeks, then take 1 week off. Best taken on empty stomach. Not for evening use.

HERBAL INSIGHts: Ginseng contains ginsenosides, compounds that help the body adapt to stress while boosting energy and mental performance. It supports healthy testosterone levels, improves circulation (important for erectile function), and enhances overall vitality. Different types have different properties—Asian is more stimulating, American more balancing.

SAFETY NOTE: *May increase blood pressure and affect blood sugar. Not for acute illness. Can interact with many medications. Start with small amounts.*

MACA ROOT FERTILITY BLEND

Incan warriors consumed maca before battle for strength and stamina. Spanish conquistadors fed it to horses to maintain fertility at high altitudes—it worked for both species!

What You'll Need:
» 1 tablespoon maca root powder
» 1 cup warm almond milk
» 1 teaspoon cacao powder
» Honey and cinnamon to taste

How to Make It:
1. Warm almond milk gently
2. Whisk in maca and cacao
3. Add honey and cinnamon
4. Blend if desired for frothiness
5. Drink immediately

Usage in Traditions: Start with 1 teaspoon daily, increase to 1 tablespoon. Take morning or afternoon. Both partners can use for fertility support.

Herbal Insights: Maca doesn't contain hormones but rather provides nutrients that support the endocrine system. It's been shown to improve sperm count and motility in men, regulate cycles in women, and boost libido in both. The root is also adaptogenic, helping bodies handle the stress that often accompanies fertility challenges.

Safety Note: *Generally safe. May affect thyroid function due to iodine content. Can cause jittery feelings if too much too fast.*

WILD YAM CREAM

Wild yam was the original source of hormones for birth control pills. Mexican women have used it for centuries for menstrual and menopausal complaints.

What You'll Need:
» 1/2 cup wild yam root infused oil
» 2 tablespoons shea butter
» 1 tablespoon beeswax
» 10 drops lavender essential oil

» 5 drops geranium essential oil

HOW TO MAKE IT:
1. Make infused oil by heating wild yam in oil 2 hours
2. Strain out root completely
3. Melt beeswax and shea butter in oil
4. Remove from heat
5. Add essential oils when cooled slightly
6. Pour into jars immediately

USAGE IN TRADITIONS: Apply 1/4 teaspoon to thin-skinned areas twice daily. Rotate sites. Use days 14-28 of cycle, or daily for menopause.

HERBAL INSIGHTS: Wild yam contains diosgenin, a precursor to progesterone. While the body can't convert it directly to progesterone, wild yam appears to support the body's own hormone production and may bind to progesterone receptors. Many women report relief from PMS, menstrual cramps, and menopausal symptoms.

SAFETY NOTE: *External use generally safe. Not a replacement for prescribed hormones. May not be appropriate for hormone-sensitive conditions.*

MOTHERWORT PMS RELIEF

The name says it all—motherwort has been women's ally for centuries. It was said to make mothers immortal, though settling for PMS relief seems more realistic!

WHAT YOU'LL NEED:
» 2 tablespoons fresh motherwort (or 1 tablespoon dried)
» 1 cup boiling water
» Honey and lemon

HOW TO MAKE IT:
1. Place motherwort in cup
2. Pour boiling water over
3. Cover and steep 15 minutes
4. Strain well
5. Add honey and lemon liberally—it's bitter!

USAGE IN TRADITIONS: Start 1 week before period: 2 cups daily. During PMS: up to 3 cups daily. Can also use tincture for convenience.

HERBAL INSIGHts: Motherwort calms the nervous system while gently supporting hormonal balance. It's particularly effective for PMS with anxiety, heart palpitations, and emotional volatility. The herb also has mild uterine tonic properties, potentially easing cramps. Its bitter compounds support liver function, helping process excess hormones.

SAFETY NOTE: *Not for pregnancy (uterine stimulant). May increase menstrual flow. Can interact with heart medications.*

ROSE HIP PREGNANCY TEA

During WWII, British children gathered rose hips for vitamin C syrup when citrus was unavailable. Pregnant women especially benefited from this nutritious "war effort."

WHAT YOU'LL NEED:
- 2 tablespoons dried rose hips
- 1 tablespoon dried hibiscus
- 1 tablespoon dried nettle
- 2 cups boiling water

HOW TO MAKE IT:
1. Combine all herbs in teapot
2. Pour boiling water over
3. Cover and steep 20 minutes
4. Strain carefully (rose hip seeds irritating)
5. Sweeten with honey if desired
6. Can drink hot or cold

USAGE IN TRADITIONS: Drink 2-3 cups daily throughout pregnancy. Especially beneficial in third trimester. Safe for entire pregnancy.

HERBAL INSIGHts: Rose hips provide gentle, food-based vitamin C essential for tissue integrity and immune function during pregnancy. Combined with mineral-rich nettle and antioxidant hibiscus, this tea provides comprehensive nutritional support. The vitamin C also enhances iron absorption—crucial during pregnancy.

SAFETY NOTE: *High vitamin C may cause loose stools in very large amounts.*

SHATAVARI WOMEN'S REJUVENATIVE

Shatavari literally means "she who has a hundred husbands"—referring to its reputation for promoting fertility and vitality. It's Ayurveda's premier women's herb.

What You'll Need:
- 1 tablespoon shatavari root powder
- 1 cup warm milk
- 1 teaspoon ghee
- Cardamom and honey to taste

How to Make It:
1. Warm milk gently
2. Add shatavari powder
3. Stir in ghee
4. Add cardamom and honey
5. Whisk until frothy
6. Drink warm

Usage in Traditions: Drink nightly for general women's health. Can increase to twice daily for specific concerns. Use consistently for best results.

Herbal Insights: Shatavari is a renowned adaptogen specifically for the female reproductive system. It contains steroidal saponins that support hormonal balance without adding hormones. The herb nourishes reproductive tissues, supports healthy menstruation, enhances fertility, and eases menopausal transition. It's also deeply nourishing, supporting overall vitality.

Safety Note: *Generally very safe. May have mild estrogenic effects. Not recommended with history of estrogen-sensitive cancers.*

CLARY SAGE HORMONE OIL

Medieval Germans added clary sage to wine, calling it "muscatel sage." It was said to induce euphoria and amorous feelings—probably why it became associated with women's health!

What You'll Need:
- 10 drops clary sage essential oil

» 5 drops geranium essential oil
» 5 drops lavender essential oil
» 2 tablespoons jojoba oil

HOW TO MAKE IT:
1. Pour jojoba oil into small dark bottle
2. Add essential oils one at a time
3. Cap and shake gently
4. Label with ingredients
5. Let synergize 24 hours before use

USAGE IN TRADITIONS: Massage into lower abdomen twice daily. Can also apply to inner ankles. Use throughout cycle or as needed for symptoms.

HERBAL INSIGHTS: Clary sage contains sclareol, which may help balance estrogen levels. When applied topically, it can help regulate menstrual cycles, ease cramps, and reduce menopausal symptoms. The oil also has antispasmodic properties for cramp relief and mood-balancing effects. Combined with hormone-balancing geranium, it creates a powerful topical remedy.

SAFETY NOTE: *Not for pregnancy or with alcohol use. Can lower blood pressure. May enhance effects of estrogen medications.*

RED CLOVER MENOPAUSE TEA

Farm animals grazing on red clover showed increased fertility, leading researchers to discover its phytoestrogen content. Wise women had been using it for "the change" all along.

WHAT YOU'LL NEED:
» 3 tablespoons dried red clover blossoms
» 1 tablespoon dried sage
» 1 tablespoon dried mint
» 1 quart boiling water

HOW TO MAKE IT:
1. Combine herbs in quart jar
2. Fill with boiling water
3. Cover and steep 4 hours or overnight
4. Strain and refrigerate
5. Drink throughout day

Usage in Traditions: Drink 2-3 cups daily for menopausal symptoms. Best used consistently for several months. Can drink hot or cold.

Herbal Insights: Red clover contains isoflavones—plant compounds that weakly mimic estrogen. These can help reduce hot flashes, night sweats, and other menopausal symptoms without the risks of hormone replacement. The addition of sage specifically targets hot flashes and night sweats, while mint improves taste and digestion.

Safety Note: *Not with blood thinners or estrogen-sensitive cancers. May affect hormone medications.*

FENUGREEK MILK SUPPLY

Egyptian women have used fenugreek to increase milk supply since ancient times. Harem women ate the seeds to enhance their curves—it builds tissue!

What You'll Need:
- 3 tablespoons fenugreek seeds
- 2 cups water
- Honey and lemon
- Fennel seeds (optional)

How to Make It:
1. Soak seeds overnight in water
2. In morning, bring to gentle boil
3. Simmer 10 minutes
4. Strain seeds (can eat them)
5. Add honey and lemon
6. Drink warm

Usage in Traditions: Drink 3 cups daily while establishing milk supply. Most women see results within 24-72 hours. Reduce once supply increases.

Herbal Insights: Fenugreek contains diosgenin, which may increase milk production. The seeds are also highly nutritious, providing vitamins and minerals depleted by breastfeeding. Many women report dramatic increases in milk supply, though the mechanism isn't fully understood. The maple syrup scent in sweat and urine indicates therapeutic dosage!

SAFETY NOTE: *Can lower blood sugar. May cause gas initially. Not for pregnancy. Allergic reactions possible in those sensitive to chickpeas.*

PYGEUM PROSTATE HEALTH

African traditional healers have used pygeum bark for "old man's disease" (enlarged prostate) for generations. European colonists learned of it and nearly drove the tree extinct through overharvesting.

WHAT YOU'LL NEED:
- » 1 tablespoon pygeum bark
- » 1 cup water
- » Saw palmetto (optional)

HOW TO MAKE IT:
1. Simmer bark in water 20 minutes
2. Cover and let cool
3. Strain thoroughly
4. Can add to saw palmetto tea
5. Drink warm or cool

USAGE IN TRADITIONS: Drink 1/2 cup twice daily with meals. Use for 2-3 months to see full effects. Can combine with other prostate herbs.

HERBAL INSIGHts: Pygeum contains phytosterols that reduce prostate inflammation and improve urinary symptoms. It specifically helps with nighttime urination, flow rate, and bladder emptying. Studies show it's particularly effective when combined with saw palmetto. The bark also has anti-inflammatory compounds that benefit overall prostate health.

SAFETY NOTE: *May cause mild stomach upset. Can interact with prostate medications.*

HORNY GOAT WEED TONIC

A Chinese goat herder noticed his flock became unusually amorous after eating this weed. He tried it himself, and horny goat weed entered the herbal pharmacy!

WHAT YOU'LL NEED:
- » 2 tablespoons horny goat weed (epimedium)

» 1 tablespoon goji berries
» 2 cups hot water
» Honey to taste

HOW TO MAKE IT:
1. Place herbs in teapot
2. Pour hot (not boiling) water over
3. Cover and steep 15 minutes
4. Strain herbs
5. Add honey if desired
6. Drink warm

USAGE IN TRADITIONS: Drink 1 cup daily, preferably in morning. Can increase to twice daily. Effects build over several weeks of use.

HERBAL INSIGHts: Horny goat weed contains icariin, a compound that may increase nitric oxide levels, improving blood flow to sexual organs. It may also support healthy testosterone levels and reduce fatigue. Despite the silly name, research confirms traditional uses for erectile dysfunction and low libido in both men and women.

SAFETY NOTE: *May affect blood pressure and heart rhythm in large doses. Not with blood thinners. Can cause dizziness or nausea if too much.*

BLUE COHOSH LABOR PREP

Native American women used blue cohosh to prepare for birth and ease labor. Midwives still use it, but with much more caution than our ancestors.

WHAT YOU'LL NEED:
» 1/2 teaspoon dried blue cohosh root
» 1 cup water
» Red raspberry leaf (to combine)

HOW TO MAKE IT:
1. Simmer blue cohosh in water 10 minutes
2. Remove from heat
3. Add raspberry leaf
4. Cover and steep 10 minutes
5. Strain carefully

Usage in Traditions: Only under supervision of qualified midwife or healthcare provider. Traditional use: 1/4 cup every 30 minutes during active labor only.

Herbal Insights: Blue cohosh contains caulosaponin, which stimulates uterine contractions. It's specifically for active labor, not pregnancy. The herb can help strengthen weak contractions and may shorten labor duration. However, it's powerful remedy requiring expertise to use safely.

Safety Note: *Potentially dangerous if misused. Can cause fetal heart problems. Only under professional supervision. Never during pregnancy.*

PARTRIDGE BERRY PREGNANCY SUPPORT

Native American women drank partridge berry tea in the final weeks of pregnancy. The berries have two "eyes" from twin flowers—symbolizing the mother-baby connection.

What You'll Need:
» 2 tablespoons dried partridge berry leaves
» 1 tablespoon red raspberry leaf
» 1 cup boiling water

How to Make It:
1. Combine herbs in teapot
2. Pour boiling water over
3. Cover and steep 20 minutes
4. Strain herbs
5. Drink warm
6. Can add honey

Usage in Traditions: Last 6 weeks of pregnancy only: 1-2 cups daily. Helps prepare uterus for birth. Safe and gentle preparation.

Herbal Insights: Partridge berry gently tones the uterus in preparation for birth without stimulating contractions. It may help prevent miscarriage when used earlier in pregnancy (under supervision). The herb also has mild diuretic properties, potentially reducing late-pregnancy swelling. Combined with raspberry leaf, it creates comprehensive uterine preparation.

Safety Note: *Consult healthcare provider for earlier use. Traditional use suggests safety but limited modern research.*

CORN SILK URINARY HEALTH

Native Americans never threw away corn silk—they knew these golden threads were remedy for urinary troubles. Waste not, want not at its finest!

What You'll Need:
» 1/4 cup fresh corn silk (or 2 tablespoons dried)
» 2 cups boiling water
» Honey to taste

How to Make It:
1. Place corn silk in teapot
2. Pour boiling water over
3. Cover and steep 15 minutes
4. Strain out silk
5. Add honey if desired
6. Drink warm or cold

Usage in Traditions: Drink 3 cups daily for urinary tract health. For acute infections, drink every 2-3 hours. Continue several days after symptoms resolve.

Herbal Insights: Corn silk is a gentle diuretic that soothes inflamed urinary tissues while increasing urine flow to flush out bacteria. It contains compounds that relax the urinary tract and may help prevent kidney stones. The silk is particularly helpful for the burning sensation of UTIs and can complement other treatments.

Safety Note: *Increases urination—stay hydrated. May affect blood sugar. Consult doctor for persistent UTIs.*

Pain and Inflammation

Pain is your body's alarm system—a signal that something needs attention. While modern medicine often seeks to silence this alarm, traditional herbalism takes a different approach: addressing the root cause while providing relief. The herbs in this chapter don't just mask pain; they reduce inflammation, improve circulation, relax muscles, and support your body's natural healing processes. From the willow bark that gave us aspirin to the exotic frankincense of ancient temples, these plants offer time-tested relief for humanity's oldest complaint.

Natural Approaches to Pain

Understanding pain helps us treat it more effectively. Acute pain—from injury or overexertion—often responds well to anti-inflammatory herbs and topical treatments. Chronic pain requires a deeper approach, addressing inflammation, tension patterns, and often emotional components. Nerve pain needs specific herbs that calm overactive nerve signals, while arthritic pain benefits from herbs that support joint health over time.

The beauty of herbal pain relief lies in its multifaceted approach. A single herb might reduce inflammation, improve circulation to affected areas, relax surrounding muscles, and lift the depression that often accompanies chronic pain. This holistic action explains why plant medicines often succeed where single-action drugs fail.

Anti-inflammatory Herbs

WILLOW BARK PAIN TEA

Hippocrates prescribed willow bark for pain 2,400 years ago. In 1897, Bayer synthesized aspirin from willow's salicin—but the whole plant remains gentler and more balanced than its famous offspring.

What You'll Need:
- » 2 tablespoons dried white willow bark
- » 1 cup water
- » Honey and lemon (optional)
- » Ginger or cinnamon for taste

How to Make It:
1. Simmer bark in water for 15 minutes
2. Cover and reduce heat to low
3. Continue simmering 5 more minutes
4. Strain out bark
5. Add honey and lemon if desired
6. Drink while warm

Usage in Traditions: Drink 1 cup every 4-6 hours for pain. Maximum 4 cups daily. For chronic pain, drink 2 cups daily regularly.

Herbal Insights: Willow bark contains salicin, which your body converts to salicylic acid—the precursor to aspirin. But unlike aspirin, willow bark also contains tannins that protect your stomach lining and flavonoids that enhance the anti-inflammatory effect. It works more slowly but more gently than aspirin, providing sustained relief without the harsh side effects.

Safety Note: *Not for those allergic to aspirin. Avoid with blood thinners or before surgery. Not for children with fever (Reye's syndrome risk).*

TURMERIC GOLDEN MILK

Indian grandmothers have served golden milk for every ache and pain for thousands of years. This "haldi doodh" is now validated by hundreds of studies showing turmeric rivals pharmaceutical anti-inflammatories.

What You'll Need:

» 1 teaspoon turmeric powder (or 1 inch fresh root)
» 1 cup milk (dairy or plant-based)
» 1/4 teaspoon black pepper
» 1/2 teaspoon coconut oil or ghee
» Honey to taste
» Pinch of cinnamon and ginger

How to Make It:
1. Warm milk gently in saucepan
2. Add turmeric and pepper
3. Whisk in oil or ghee
4. Simmer 5 minutes, whisking frequently
5. Strain if using fresh root
6. Add honey and spices

Usage in Traditions: Drink 1-2 cups daily for chronic inflammation. For acute pain, drink 3 times daily. Best absorbed with fat and black pepper.

Herbal Insights: Turmeric's curcumin is one of nature's most powerful anti-inflammatories, blocking the same pathways as ibuprofen but without damaging your gut. The black pepper increases absorption by 2000%, while the fat helps this fat-soluble compound enter your cells. Regular use reduces systemic inflammation, easing everything from arthritis to post-workout soreness.

Safety Note: *May increase bleeding risk. Can lower blood sugar. Large amounts may cause digestive upset. May interact with blood thinners.*

DEVIL'S CLAW JOINT RELIEF

African San people have used devil's claw for centuries, especially for joint pain. The name comes from its vicious-looking seed pods—but the root has beneficial properties.

What You'll Need:
» 1 teaspoon dried devil's claw root
» 1 cup boiling water
» Honey to mask bitterness

How to Make It:
1. Place root in cup or teapot
2. Pour boiling water over

3. Cover and steep 15 minutes
4. Strain thoroughly
5. Add honey liberally—it's very bitter

USAGE IN TRADITIONS: Drink 1 cup twice daily for arthritis. Best taken regularly for 4-8 weeks to see full effects. Can also use standardized extracts.

HERBAL INSIGHTS: Devil's claw contains harpagoside, a compound that reduces inflammation specifically in joints and connective tissue. Studies show it can be as effective as conventional arthritis drugs for reducing pain and improving mobility. It seems to work by blocking inflammatory enzymes while supporting cartilage health.

SAFETY NOTE: *May increase stomach acid. Not with ulcers or gallstones. Can affect heart rhythm and blood pressure. Avoid with blood thinners.*

GINGER COMPRESS

Chinese medicine has used ginger compresses for 5,000 years. Warriors applied them before battle to prevent injury and after to speed healing—external and internal fire.

WHAT YOU'LL NEED:
» 3 inch piece fresh ginger root
» 2 cups water
» Clean cloth or small towel
» Plastic wrap
» Larger towel for covering

HOW TO MAKE IT:
1. Grate ginger finely
2. Simmer in water 10 minutes
3. Strain, keeping liquid hot
4. Soak cloth in ginger water
5. Wring out excess (use gloves—it's hot!)
6. Apply to painful area immediately

USAGE IN TRADITIONS: Apply hot compress for 20-30 minutes. Cover with plastic wrap then towel to retain heat. Repeat 2-3 times daily for acute pain.

HERBAL INSIGHTS: Ginger's warming compounds penetrate deeply, increasing circulation to bring healing blood flow while carrying away inflammatory waste products. The heat and ginger work synergistically—the warmth opens pores for better absorption while ginger's anti-inflammatory compounds reduce pain and stiffness. It's particularly effective for chronic, cold-type pain that feels better with warmth.

SAFETY NOTE: *Test temperature carefully to avoid burns. May cause skin irritation in sensitive individuals. Not for acute injuries with swelling.*

BOSWELLIA ANTI-INFLAMMATORY

Frankincense was worth more than gold in ancient times. The Magi brought it to baby Jesus, but they probably should have saved some for Mary's post-birth recovery!

WHAT YOU'LL NEED:
- 1 teaspoon boswellia resin tears (or powder)
- 1 cup hot water
- Honey and lemon

HOW TO MAKE IT:
1. Crush resin tears into powder if needed
2. Add to hot (not boiling) water
3. Stir vigorously—resin doesn't dissolve easily
4. Let steep 10 minutes, stirring occasionally
5. Strain if needed
6. Add honey and lemon

USAGE IN TRADITIONS: Drink 1-2 cups daily for inflammatory conditions. Can also take standardized extracts. Best with food to improve absorption.

HERBAL INSIGHTS: Boswellia contains boswellic acids that inhibit 5-LOX, an enzyme that produces inflammatory compounds. Unlike NSAIDs, it doesn't damage your stomach lining or kidneys. It's particularly effective for inflammatory arthritis, inflammatory bowel disease, and asthma. The resin also supports healthy circulation to affected areas.

Safety Note: *Generally very safe. May cause digestive upset in some. Can interact with auto-immune medications.*

MEADOWSWEET PAIN TEA

Queen Elizabeth I had meadowsweet strewn on palace floors—its sweet scent masked odors while its compounds may have reduced palace inhabitants' aches and pains through aromatherapy!

What You'll Need:
» 2 tablespoons dried meadowsweet flowers and leaves
» 1 cup boiling water
» Honey to taste

How to Make It:
1. Place meadowsweet in teapot
2. Pour boiling water over herbs
3. Cover and steep 15 minutes
4. Strain herbs
5. Add honey if desired
6. Drink warm

Usage in Traditions: Drink 1 cup up to 4 times daily for pain and inflammation. Especially good for headaches and digestive pain.

Herbal Insights: Meadowsweet contains natural salicylates like aspirin, but also has tannins and mucilage that protect your stomach—solving aspirin's main side effect. It's particularly good for pain with an inflammatory component, including headaches, arthritis, and muscle aches. The herb also helps with acid reflux, making it perfect for those who can't tolerate other pain remedies.

Safety Note: *Avoid if allergic to aspirin, though reactions are rare. Not for children with fever.*

CAYENNE PAIN SALVE

Native Americans knew that pepper could paradoxically relieve pain. They called it "cayenne" from the Tupi word "kyinha".

What You'll Need:
» 1/4 cup cayenne pepper powder

» 1 cup olive oil
» 2 ounces beeswax
» 10 drops peppermint essential oil
» 10 drops camphor essential oil
» Gloves for preparation

How to Make It:
1. Wear gloves throughout!
2. Gently warm oil and cayenne 2 hours
3. Strain through fine mesh
4. Return oil to heat, add beeswax
5. Once melted, remove from heat
6. Add essential oils
7. Pour into tins immediately

Usage in Traditions: Apply small amount to painful areas 2-3 times daily. Always wash hands thoroughly after. Avoid face and sensitive areas.

Herbal Insights: Cayenne's capsaicin depletes substance P, the neurotransmitter that signals pain to your brain. First it causes warming and mild burning, then numbness, then long-lasting pain relief. It also dramatically increases blood flow to the area, bringing healing nutrients and removing inflammatory compounds. This double action makes it incredibly effective for arthritis, neuropathy, and muscle pain.

Safety Note: *Will burn sensitive skin. Never use on broken skin. Keep away from children and pets. Always label clearly.*

WHITE WILLOW HEADACHE TEA

Ancient Egyptians chewed willow leaves for headaches. The Ebers Papyrus from 1534 BCE mentions willow for pain—making this one of humanity's oldest documented remedies.

What You'll Need:
» 1 tablespoon white willow bark
» 1 teaspoon feverfew leaves
» 1 cup water
» Peppermint and honey (optional)

How to Make It:

1. Simmer willow bark in water 10 minutes
2. Add feverfew leaves
3. Remove from heat and steep 10 minutes
4. Strain herbs
5. Add peppermint and honey
6. Drink warm

Usage in Traditions: Drink at first sign of headache. Can repeat every 4 hours. For chronic headaches, drink 1-2 cups daily preventively.

Herbal Insights: White willow provides gentle aspirin-like compounds while feverfew prevents migraine by inhibiting inflammatory prostaglandins and preventing platelet aggregation. Together they address both tension and vascular headaches. The addition of peppermint provides aromatherapy benefits and helps with any associated nausea.

Safety Note: *Not for aspirin allergy or children with fever. Feverfew can cause mouth irritation. Avoid before surgery.*

CAT'S CLAW ARTHRITIS SUPPORT

Peruvian Asháninka people have used cat's claw for thousands of years. They say the spirit of the jaguar lives in the vine—giving it power over inflammation and pain.

What You'll Need:
» 1 tablespoon cat's claw bark
» 1 cup water
» Lemon juice
» Honey (optional)

How to Make It:
1. Add bark to cold water
2. Bring to gentle simmer
3. Simmer 15 minutes covered
4. Strain bark
5. Add lemon juice
6. Sweeten if desired

Usage in Traditions: Drink 1 cup twice daily between meals. Use for 8-12 weeks then take a break. Can also use standardized extracts.

HERBAL INSIGHts: Cat's claw contains unique alkaloids that reduce inflammation and modulate immune function—perfect for autoimmune arthritis. It inhibits TNF-alpha, a major inflammatory cytokine, while supporting overall joint health. The vine also has antioxidant properties that protect joints from further damage.

SAFETY NOTE: *May slow blood clotting. Not with immune-suppressing drugs or before surgery. Can lower blood pressure.*

FEVERFEW MIGRAINE PREVENTION

Medieval physicians called it "featherfew" for its feathery leaves. Women would eat a leaf wrapped in bread daily to prevent "megrim"—their term for migraine.

WHAT YOU'LL NEED:
» 2-3 fresh feverfew leaves (or 1 teaspoon dried)
» Bread or honey to mask bitterness
» Cup of water if making tea

HOW TO MAKE IT:
1. For fresh: sandwich leaves in bread
2. For tea: steep dried leaves 10 minutes
3. Strain if making tea
4. Add honey to mask bitter taste
5. Consume immediately

USAGE IN TRADITIONS: Eat 2-3 fresh leaves daily (or drink 1 cup tea) for prevention. Must use daily for 4-6 weeks to see effects. Not for acute migraines.

HERBAL INSIGHts: Feverfew contains parthenolide, which prevents the cascade of inflammatory events that trigger migraines. It inhibits prostaglandin synthesis and prevents platelet aggregation—addressing multiple migraine mechanisms. Regular use can reduce frequency, severity, and duration of migraines. Studies show it's as effective as some prescription preventives.

SAFETY NOTE: *Can cause mouth ulcers. Not during pregnancy. Don't stop suddenly after long use—taper off. May increase bleeding.*

JAMAICA DOGWOOD NERVE PAIN

Caribbean fishermen threw Jamaica dogwood bark in tidal pools to stun fish. Healers recognized that what calms fish nerves might help human nerve pain—they were right!

What You'll Need:
» 1 teaspoon Jamaica dogwood bark
» 1 cup water
» Valerian or passionflower (optional)
» Honey to taste

How to Make It:
1. Simmer bark in water 15 minutes
2. Cover and reduce heat
3. Continue simmering 5 minutes
4. Strain bark
5. Add honey
6. Drink warm before bed

Usage in Traditions: Drink 1/2 cup for nerve pain, especially at bedtime. Can take up to 2 cups daily. Best for short-term use.

Herbal Insights: Jamaica dogwood contains compounds that specifically calm overactive nerves, making it invaluable for neuralgia, sciatica, and nerve-related insomnia. It's both analgesic and sedative, addressing the pain that keeps you awake. Unlike opiates, it's not addictive, though it should still be used judiciously.

Safety Note: *Potent herb—don't exceed recommended dose. Can cause nausea in large amounts. Not for pregnancy or with sedatives.*

CORYDALIS PAIN TINCTURE

Traditional Chinese Medicine has used corydalis (yan hu suo) for pain relief for over 1,000 years. It's said to "move blood and stop pain"—especially menstrual and trauma pain.

What You'll Need:
» 1/2 cup dried corydalis root
» 1 1/2 cups vodka
» Glass jar with lid
» Amber bottles for storage

HOW TO MAKE IT:
1. Grind corydalis root coarsely
2. Place in jar and cover with vodka
3. Shake well and cap tightly
4. Store in dark place 6 weeks
5. Shake daily first week
6. Strain and bottle in amber glass

USAGE IN TRADITIONS: Take 30-60 drops in water for pain. Can take every 4 hours as needed. Especially effective for menstrual cramps and trauma.

HERBAL INSIGHtS: Corydalis contains tetrahydropalmatine (THP), an alkaloid that's been called "nature's morphine"—though much gentler and non-addictive. It blocks pain signals in the brain while promoting circulation to injured areas. It's particularly effective for sharp, stabbing pains and pain that worsens with pressure.

SAFETY NOTE: *Don't use with MAO inhibitors or sedatives. May cause drowsiness. Not for pregnancy or liver disease.*

PINE BARK JOINT SUPPORT

Jacques Cartier's crew survived scurvy in 1536 thanks to Native Americans' pine bark tea. The same compounds that saved sailors now help aging joints!

WHAT YOU'LL NEED:
- 2 tablespoons pine bark (or maritime pine extract)
- 2 cups water
- Honey and lemon

HOW TO MAKE IT:
1. Simmer pine bark in water 20 minutes
2. Cover and let steep additional 20 minutes
3. Strain out bark
4. Add honey and lemon
5. Can drink hot or cold

USAGE IN TRADITIONS: Drink 1-2 cups daily for joint health. Standardized extracts (Pycnogenol) also available. Best with consistent use.

HERBAL INSIGHTS: Pine bark contains oligomeric proanthocyanidins (OPCs), powerful antioxidants that reduce inflammation and support collagen production. These compounds specifically benefit joint health by protecting cartilage from breakdown while promoting repair. Studies show improvement in joint pain, stiffness, and function.

SAFETY NOTE: *May increase immune function—caution with autoimmune conditions. Can lower blood sugar.*

CELERY SEED GOUT RELIEF

Ancient Romans wore celery wreaths to prevent hangovers—which often triggered gout attacks. They were onto something: celery seed remains one of the best gout remedies.

WHAT YOU'LL NEED:
» 1 tablespoon celery seeds
» 1 cup boiling water
» Honey (optional)

HOW TO MAKE IT:
1. Crush celery seeds lightly
2. Place in cup or teapot
3. Pour boiling water over
4. Cover and steep 15 minutes
5. Strain seeds
6. Add honey if desired

USAGE IN TRADITIONS: Drink 2-3 cups daily during gout flares. For prevention, drink 1 cup daily. Can also take standardized extracts.

HERBAL INSIGHTS: Celery seeds help eliminate uric acid, the crystal-forming compound that causes gout's excruciating pain. They're also anti-inflammatory and mildly diuretic, helping flush out the problematic crystals. The seeds contain 3-n-butylphthalide, which specifically reduces inflammation in joints.

SAFETY NOTE: *May increase photosensitivity. Not during pregnancy in medicinal amounts. Can interact with thyroid medications.*

BUTTERBUR MIGRAINE TEA

Medieval Europeans wrapped butter in butterbur's huge leaves—hence the name. They also used it for plague and fever, but we now know it excels at preventing migraines.

What You'll Need:
» Standardized butterbur extract (PA-free only)
» Or 1 teaspoon dried butterbur root (properly processed)
» 1 cup hot water

How to Make It:
1. Use only PA-free standardized extracts
2. Follow package directions precisely
3. If using processed root, steep 10 minutes
4. Strain carefully
5. Don't exceed recommended amounts

Usage in Traditions: Take standardized extract as directed (usually 75mg twice daily). For prevention only—not acute treatment. Use for 4-6 months.

Herbal Insights: Butterbur contains petasin and isopetasin, compounds that reduce inflammation and prevent blood vessel spasms associated with migraines. Clinical trials show it can reduce migraine frequency by up to 50%. It works preventively by stabilizing blood vessel reactivity and reducing inflammatory responses.

Safety Note: *Only use products certified PA-free (toxic alkaloids removed). Can cause digestive upset. Not for pregnancy or liver disease.*

BIRCH BARK MUSCLE RUB

Native Americans taught colonists to use birch bark for pain. Its wintergreen scent comes from the same compound—methyl salicylate—used in commercial muscle rubs.

What You'll Need:
» 1/2 cup birch bark (black or yellow birch)
» 1 cup oil (olive or sweet almond)
» 1 ounce beeswax
» 20 drops peppermint essential oil

HOW TO MAKE IT:
1. Infuse birch bark in oil using double boiler 2 hours
2. Strain out bark completely
3. Return oil to heat, add beeswax
4. Stir until melted
5. Remove from heat, add peppermint oil
6. Pour into containers

USAGE IN TRADITIONS: Massage into sore muscles 2-3 times daily. Excellent for post-exercise soreness or chronic muscle pain.

HERBAL INSIGHTS: Birch bark contains natural methyl salicylate, which penetrates skin to reduce inflammation and pain in muscles and joints. It increases local blood flow, helping flush out lactic acid and inflammatory compounds. The warming sensation also confuses pain signals, providing immediate relief while the anti-inflammatory compounds work deeper.

SAFETY NOTE: *Contains natural aspirin compounds—not for aspirin allergy. Don't use on broken skin. Keep away from children.*

YUCCA JOINT TEA

Southwestern Native Americans called yucca "soap plant" and used it for everything from shampoo to arthritis. The same saponins that make it sudsy also reduce inflammation.

WHAT YOU'LL NEED:
» 1 tablespoon dried yucca root
» 1 cup water
» Honey and lemon

HOW TO MAKE IT:
1. Simmer yucca root in water 15 minutes
2. Cover and let cool
3. Strain root
4. Add honey and lemon
5. Drink warm or cold

USAGE IN TRADITIONS: Drink 1/2 cup twice daily for joint pain. Start slowly—can cause digestive upset. Use for 4-6 weeks then take break.

HERBAL INSIGHts: Yucca contains steroidal saponins that have cortisone-like anti-inflammatory effects without the side effects. These compounds reduce joint inflammation and may help rebuild cartilage. Some people experience dramatic improvement in arthritis symptoms, possibly due to yucca's ability to improve fat absorption and reduce endotoxins.

SAFETY NOTE: *Start with small amounts—can cause digestive upset. May affect fat-soluble vitamin absorption with long-term use.*

CLOVE TOOTHACHE OIL

Chinese dentists used clove oil 2,000 years ago. Until modern anesthetics, it was dentistry's main pain reliever—and it still works when you can't get to the dentist!

WHAT YOU'LL NEED:
- 10 whole cloves (or clove essential oil)
- 1 tablespoon olive oil
- Small dark bottle
- Cotton swabs for application

HOW TO MAKE IT:
1. If using whole cloves, crush lightly
2. Place in small jar with olive oil
3. Let infuse 24 hours
4. Strain and bottle
5. Or mix 5 drops clove oil with 1 tablespoon olive oil

USAGE IN TRADITIONS: Apply drop directly to affected tooth with cotton swab. Can reapply every 2-3 hours. See dentist as soon as possible.

HERBAL INSIGHts: Clove contains eugenol, a powerful anesthetic and antiseptic. It numbs pain on contact while fighting infection—addressing both symptoms and cause. Eugenol is so effective it's still used in professional dental preparations. The oil also reduces inflammation and promotes healing.

SAFETY NOTE: *Can burn soft tissues—apply only to tooth. Not for children under 2. Temporary relief only—see dentist.*

BLACK PEPPER WARMING OIL

Black pepper was once worth its weight in gold. Roman soldiers received pepper rations, and medieval rents were paid in peppercorns—this "black gold" warmed bodies and relieved pain.

What You'll Need:
- 2 tablespoons black peppercorns
- 1 cup sesame or mustard oil
- 1 tablespoon dried ginger
- Glass jar for infusing

How to Make It:
1. Coarsely grind peppercorns
2. Add to oil with ginger
3. Warm gently 1 hour (don't overheat)
4. Let cool and infuse 48 hours
5. Strain through fine mesh
6. Store in dark bottle

Usage in Traditions: Massage into stiff, cold, achy areas. Excellent for morning stiffness or chronic pain that worsens with cold.

Herbal Insights: Black pepper's piperine increases circulation and enhances absorption of other compounds. It creates warming sensations that relax muscles and confuse pain signals. The oil is particularly effective for "cold" type pain—stiffness that improves with movement and warmth. It also has mild analgesic properties.

Safety Note: *Can irritate sensitive skin—dilute more if needed. Not for inflamed or hot conditions. Patch test first.*

FRANKINCENSE JOINT CREAM

Egyptian pharaohs burned a fortune in frankincense daily. While they sought divine favor, they inadvertently inhaled powerful anti-inflammatory compounds—explaining their legendary longevity!

What You'll Need:
- 1/2 cup shea butter
- 1/4 cup coconut oil
- 20 drops frankincense essential oil
- 10 drops myrrh essential oil

» 10 drops ginger essential oil

HOW TO MAKE IT:
1. Melt shea butter and coconut oil together
2. Remove from heat and cool slightly
3. Add essential oils
4. Whip with mixer until fluffy
5. Transfer to jars
6. Let set at room temperature

USAGE IN TRADITIONS: Massage into painful joints 2-3 times daily. Especially good for arthritis and old injuries. Use regularly for best results.

HERBAL INSIGHts: Frankincense contains boswellic acids that inhibit inflammatory enzymes, particularly 5-LOX. When applied topically, these compounds penetrate to reduce joint inflammation and pain. The addition of myrrh enhances anti-inflammatory effects while ginger increases circulation. This combination addresses pain, inflammation, and stiffness simultaneously.

SAFETY NOTE: *Some people sensitive to essential oils—patch test. Not for broken skin.*

ANGELICA CIRCULATION OIL

Legend says an angel revealed this plant's medicinal properties during a plague—hence "angelica." Whether divine or not, it definitely gets blood moving to painful areas.

WHAT YOU'LL NEED:
» 1/4 cup dried angelica root
» 1 cup olive oil
» 10 drops rosemary essential oil
» 5 drops black pepper essential oil

HOW TO MAKE IT:
1. Infuse angelica in oil using double boiler 2 hours
2. Strain out root material
3. Let cool to room temperature
4. Add essential oils
5. Bottle in dark glass
6. Label with ingredients

Usage in Traditions: Massage into areas with poor circulation or chronic pain. Excellent for cold hands/feet and pain that worsens with cold.

Herbal INSIGHts: Angelica is a powerful circulatory stimulant, bringing fresh blood to areas that need healing. It contains coumarins that dilate blood vessels and phthalides that relax smooth muscle. This increased circulation helps remove inflammatory compounds while delivering nutrients for repair. It's particularly good for chronic pain with a cold, stagnant quality.

Safety Note: *Photosensitizing—avoid sun exposure on treated areas. Not during pregnancy. May interact with blood thinners.*

WILD YAM ANTISPASMODIC

Aztec women used wild yam for menstrual cramps and childbirth. It later became the source for synthetic hormones, but the whole plant offers gentle relief without side effects.

What You'll Need:
» 2 tablespoons dried wild yam root
» 1 cup water
» Cramp bark (optional addition)
» Honey to taste

How to Make It:
1. Simmer wild yam in water 20 minutes
2. Add cramp bark last 10 minutes if using
3. Cover and let cool
4. Strain herbs
5. Add honey
6. Drink warm

Usage in Traditions: Drink 1/2 cup every 2-3 hours for cramps and spasms. Especially effective for menstrual and intestinal cramps.

Herbal INSIGHts: Wild yam contains diosgenin and other compounds that relax smooth muscle, making it excellent for cramps anywhere in the body. It's particularly effective for menstrual cramps, intestinal spasms, and gallbladder pain. The antispasmodic effect is gentle but reliable, without the drowsiness of pharmaceutical muscle relaxants.

Safety Note: *Not the same as progesterone despite marketing claims. Avoid during pregnancy.*

KAVA MUSCLE RELAXER

Pacific islanders say kava was given by the gods to resolve conflicts peacefully. When your muscles are in conflict with relaxation, kava brings divine intervention!

What You'll Need:
- 2 tablespoons kava root powder
- 1 cup warm water
- Coconut milk (optional)
- Strainer bag

How to Make It:
1. Place kava in strainer bag
2. Put in bowl with warm water
3. Knead bag for 10 minutes
4. Water should turn cloudy brown
5. Add coconut milk if desired
6. Drink immediately

Usage in Traditions: Drink 1/2 cup for muscle tension. Can repeat in 30 minutes. Especially good for tension from stress or anxiety.

Herbal Insights: Kava contains kavalactones that relax muscles through multiple mechanisms—they enhance GABA activity, block sodium channels, and reduce nerve excitation. The result is profound muscle relaxation without weakness or impairment. It's particularly effective for psychosomatic muscle tension—when stress literally ties you in knots.

Safety Note: *Use only water-based preparations. Don't combine with alcohol or sedatives. May affect liver with poor quality or excessive use.*

BLUE COHOSH CRAMPING

Native American women used blue cohosh specifically for childbirth and menstrual issues. Unlike its cousin black cohosh, blue cohosh is powerful medicine requiring respect and knowledge.

What You'll Need:
- 1/2 teaspoon dried blue cohosh root
- 1 cup water
- Wild yam or cramp bark (safer additions)

How to Make It:
1. Simmer blue cohosh in water 10 minutes
2. Use minimal amounts—it's potent
3. Combine with gentler herbs
4. Strain carefully
5. Use with caution

Usage in Traditions: Only under professional guidance. Traditional use for severe cramping, but safer alternatives usually preferred.

Herbal Insights: Blue cohosh contains caulosaponin, which powerfully affects smooth muscle. It can relieve severe cramping but must be used carefully. The compounds specifically target uterine and intestinal smooth muscle, making it effective but potentially dangerous if misused.

Safety Note: *Potentially dangerous herb. Can cause serious side effects. Only under professional supervision. Many safer alternatives available.*

WINTERGREEN PAIN OIL

Revolutionary War soldiers chewed wintergreen leaves to prevent scurvy and relieve pain. The same compound that freshens breath also penetrates deeply to relieve pain.

What You'll Need:
- 20 drops wintergreen essential oil
- 1/4 cup carrier oil
- 10 drops peppermint oil
- Dark glass bottle

How to Make It:

1. Mix carrier oil in bottle
2. Add wintergreen oil drop by drop
3. Add peppermint oil
4. Cap and shake well
5. Label clearly—this is potent
6. Let synergize 24 hours

USAGE IN TRADITIONS: Apply small amount to painful areas 2-3 times daily. Excellent for muscle pain, arthritis, and neuralgia. Wash hands after use.

HERBAL INSIGHts: Wintergreen oil is nearly pure methyl salicylate—natural aspirin that penetrates skin to reduce inflammation and pain. It increases local blood flow while blocking pain signals. The addition of peppermint creates a cooling sensation that enhances pain relief. This combination provides both immediate relief and longer-term anti-inflammatory effects.

SAFETY NOTE: *Never use undiluted. Toxic if ingested. Not for children, pregnancy, or aspirin allergy. Can be absorbed through skin—don't overuse.*

Children's Gentle Herbs

Little ones experience big discomforts in small bodies. From teething pain to tummy troubles, children face many of the same ailments as adults but require gentler approaches. The remedies in this chapter have soothed fussy babies and comforted sick children for generations, using herbs so mild that even the most delicate systems can benefit.

Special Considerations for Children

Children aren't simply small adults—their bodies process herbs differently, requiring adjusted dosages and gentler preparations. Their developing systems respond more sensitively to plant medicines, which can be both a blessing and a caution.

When preparing remedies for children, taste matters immensely. The most effective herb won't help if a child refuses to take it. That's why traditional children's remedies often incorporate honey (for children over one year), glycerin, or naturally sweet herbs. Many preparations can be made into popsicles, gummies, or mixed into favorite foods.

Dosage for children typically follows Clark's Rule: divide the child's weight by 150, then multiply the adult dose by this fraction. For example, a 50-pound child would take 1/3 the adult dose. However, with gentle herbs like chamomile or catnip, precise dosing is less critical. Start with less and increase as needed.

Safety remains paramount. While the herbs in this chapter have been used safely for centuries, always introduce new herbs one at a time to watch for reactions. Avoid strong herbs, essential oils (unless specifically indicated), and anything with known toxicity. When in doubt, consult with a healthcare provider familiar with herbal medicine. Remember, herbs support health but serious conditions require professional medical attention.

Kid-Friendly Herbal Support

CHAMOMILE TEETHING TEA

Peter Rabbit's mother knew best when she gave him chamomile tea. European mothers have relied on this gentle flower for teething babies since Roman times, often soaking bread in the tea for babies to gnaw.

What You'll Need:
- 1 tablespoon dried chamomile flowers
- 1 cup boiling water
- Clean washcloth for topical use

How to Make It:
1. Pour boiling water over chamomile
2. Cover and steep 10 minutes
3. Strain carefully when cool
4. For topical use, soak washcloth in tea
5. Refrigerate soaked cloth for extra relief

Usage in Traditions: For babies 6+ months: Give 1-2 teaspoons of room temperature tea up to 4 times daily. Can also let baby chew on cold, tea-soaked washcloth.

Herbal Insights: Chamomile contains compounds that reduce inflammation and pain while calming fussy babies. Its mild sedative effect helps with the irritability that accompanies teething. When applied topically via a cold washcloth, it numbs sore gums while the cold reduces swelling.

Safety Note: *Very rare allergic reactions in daisy-sensitive individuals. Start with small amounts. Always supervise when giving baby something to chew.*

CATNIP COLIC RELIEF

While cats go wild for catnip, it has the opposite effect on humans. Pioneer mothers grew it specifically for colicky babies, calling it "infant's friend."

What You'll Need:

» 1 teaspoon dried catnip
» 1 cup boiling water
» Honey (only for babies over 1 year)

HOW TO MAKE IT:
1. Pour boiling water over catnip
2. Cover and steep 5 minutes only
3. Strain while warm
4. Cool to room temperature
5. Add honey if age-appropriate

USAGE IN TRADITIONS: Newborns: 1/2 teaspoon as needed. 6+ months: 1-2 teaspoons. Toddlers: 1-2 tablespoons. Can give up to 4 times daily for colic or upset stomach.

HERBAL INSIGHts: Catnip gently relaxes intestinal spasms while calming the nervous system. It's particularly effective for colic because it addresses both the physical discomfort and the distress it causes. The herb also helps expel gas, often the culprit in infant crying.

SAFETY NOTE: *Start with small amounts to ensure tolerance. May cause drowsiness—perfect for bedtime.*

ELDERFLOWER FEVER TEA

European children were given elderflower tea to "sweat out" fevers. Unlike fever suppressants, it supports the body's natural healing process while keeping children comfortable.

WHAT YOU'LL NEED:
» 2 tablespoons dried elderflowers
» 1 tablespoon peppermint (for older children)
» 1 cup boiling water
» Honey (for children over 1)

HOW TO MAKE IT:
1. Combine herbs in teapot
2. Pour boiling water over
3. Cover and steep 10 minutes
4. Strain when lukewarm
5. Sweeten if appropriate

Usage in Traditions: Give warm (not hot) in small frequent sips. Under 2: 1-2 teaspoons every hour. Over 2: 1/4 cup every 2 hours. Continue until fever breaks naturally.

Herbal Insights: Elderflower is a gentle diaphoretic—it promotes sweating to cool the body naturally. Unlike medications that suppress fever, it works with the body's immune response. The flowers also have antiviral properties and reduce respiratory congestion often accompanying fevers.

Safety Note: *Supports natural fever process. Always monitor fever and seek medical care for high fevers, babies under 3 months, or concerning symptoms.*

LEMON BALM TUMMY TEA

Medieval monks grew lemon balm in monastery gardens specifically for children's ailments. They called it "heart's delight" for its ability to cheer up sick little ones.

What You'll Need:
- 2 tablespoons fresh lemon balm (or 1 tablespoon dried)
- 1 cup hot water
- Honey to taste (if over 1 year)

How to Make It:
1. Pour hot water over lemon balm
2. Cover to preserve volatile oils
3. Steep 10 minutes
4. Strain and cool to lukewarm
5. Sweeten if desired

Usage in Traditions: For upset stomach: 1-3 teaspoons for babies, 1/4 cup for toddlers, 1/2 cup for older children. Can give every 2-3 hours as needed.

Herbal Insights: Lemon balm calms both digestive and nervous systems—perfect for tummy aches caused by worry or excitement. It relieves gas, reduces spasms, and has mild antiviral properties. The pleasant lemony taste makes it easy to administer.

Safety Note: *Extremely safe. May cause mild drowsiness. No known contraindications for children.*

DILL SEED GRIPE WATER

Victorian nannies always kept gripe water on hand. The original recipes contained alcohol, but this traditional version uses only dill and fennel—just as effective without the concerns.

WHAT YOU'LL NEED:
- 1 teaspoon dill seeds
- 1 teaspoon fennel seeds
- 1 cup boiling water

HOW TO MAKE IT:
1. Lightly crush seeds
2. Pour boiling water over seeds
3. Cover and steep 15 minutes
4. Strain through fine mesh
5. Cool completely before use

USAGE IN TRADITIONS: Newborns: 1/2 teaspoon before feeds. Older babies: 1-2 teaspoons as needed. Can give up to 6 times daily for gas and colic.

HERBAL INSIGHTS: Dill and fennel seeds contain volatile oils that relax intestinal spasms and help expel gas. They also have mild antimicrobial properties that can help with digestive upset. This traditional combination has soothed gassy babies for centuries.

SAFETY NOTE: *Rare allergic reactions possible. If colic persists, consult healthcare provider.*

CALENDULA DIAPER CREAM

Medieval mothers called calendula "Mary's gold" and used it for all baby skin troubles. It was often the first herb planted in a garden after a baby's birth.

WHAT YOU'LL NEED:
- 1/2 cup calendula-infused oil
- 2 tablespoons beeswax
- 1 tablespoon zinc oxide powder
- 5 drops lavender essential oil (optional)

HOW TO MAKE IT:

1. Gently heat infused oil and beeswax until melted
2. Remove from heat
3. Whisk in zinc oxide carefully
4. Add lavender oil if using
5. Pour into containers immediately

USAGE IN TRADITIONS: Apply liberally with each diaper change. Can use preventatively or to treat existing rash. Safe for cloth diapers.

HERBAL INSIGHts: Calendula reduces inflammation and fights infection while promoting skin healing. Zinc oxide creates a protective barrier against moisture. The combination soothes angry skin while preventing further irritation—addressing both cause and symptoms of diaper rash.

SAFETY NOTE: *Very safe. Test on small area first. Discontinue if rash worsens—may need medical evaluation.*

MARSHMALLOW SORE THROAT POPS

Before marshmallows became sugary treats, they were medicine. French confectioners originally made pâte de guimauve (marshmallow paste) to soothe children's sore throats.

WHAT YOU'LL NEED:
» 2 tablespoons marshmallow root
» 1 cup water
» 1/4 cup honey (if over 1 year)
» Popsicle molds

HOW TO MAKE IT:
1. Simmer marshmallow root in water 20 minutes
2. Strain, pressing out mucilage
3. Add honey while warm
4. Cool completely
5. Pour into popsicle molds
6. Freeze until solid

USAGE IN TRADITIONS: Let child suck on popsicle as needed for sore throat relief. Can have 3-4 per day during illness.

HERBAL INSIGHts: Marshmallow root creates a soothing mucilage that coats inflamed throat tissues. When frozen, it provides numbing relief while the coating action continues as it melts. Kids think they're getting a treat while receiving effective medicine.

SAFETY NOTE: *Supervise young children with popsicles. Not for babies under 1 if using honey.*

OAT STRAW BATH

Farm children with the softest skin often helped with oat harvesting. Mothers noticed and began adding oat straw to baths for children with irritated skin.

WHAT YOU'LL NEED:
- 1 cup oat straw (or rolled oats)
- Large muslin bag or clean sock
- Warm bath water

HOW TO MAKE IT:
1. Fill muslin bag with oat straw
2. Tie securely
3. Place in bath while filling
4. Squeeze bag occasionally to release milk
5. Let child play with bag in tub

USAGE IN TRADITIONS: Let child soak 15-20 minutes. Can use daily for skin conditions. Pat dry gently—don't rinse off oat residue.

HERBAL INSIGHTS: Oats contain compounds that reduce skin inflammation and itching. The proteins and lipids form a protective barrier on skin while the avenanthramides specifically combat irritation. It's effective for eczema, chicken pox, and general dry skin.

SAFETY NOTE: *Ensure water temperature appropriate. Rare oat allergies possible.*

LAVENDER SLEEP DROPS

Victorian nurseries always had lavender sachets. Nannies knew that babies slept better surrounded by its gentle scent—now confirmed by sleep studies.

WHAT YOU'LL NEED:
- 1/4 cup dried lavender flowers

» 1 cup boiling water
» Vegetable glycerin
» Dropper bottle

HOW TO MAKE IT:
1. Make strong lavender tea
2. Steep covered 20 minutes
3. Strain and measure liquid
4. Add equal amount glycerin
5. Mix well and bottle

USAGE IN TRADITIONS: 6-12 months: 5 drops in water before bed. Toddlers: 10 drops. Older children: 15-20 drops. Can also add to bath.

HERBAL INSIGHTS: Lavender promotes relaxation through multiple pathways—its compounds affect GABA receptors while the scent directly impacts the limbic system. The glycerin preserves the remedy while adding sweetness kids enjoy.

SAFETY NOTE: *Some find lavender stimulating—discontinue if child becomes more active.*

FENNEL HONEY COUGH SYRUP

Greek mothers gave their children fennel honey for coughs, knowing it would soothe throats while helping expel mucus. The sweet licorice flavor made it beloved medicine.

WHAT YOU'LL NEED:
» 2 tablespoons fennel seeds
» 1 cup water
» 1/2 cup honey (over 1 year only)
» Lemon juice (optional)

HOW TO MAKE IT:
1. Simmer fennel seeds in water 15 minutes
2. Strain while hot
3. Measure liquid, add equal amount honey
4. Warm gently to combine
5. Add lemon juice if desired
6. Store refrigerated

USAGE IN TRADITIONS: 1-3 years: 1/2 teaspoon every 4 hours. 3-6 years: 1 teaspoon. Over 6: 2 teaspoons. Maximum 4 doses daily.

HERBAL INSIGHTS: Fennel acts as an expectorant, helping thin and expel mucus while soothing spasmodic coughs. The seeds' antimicrobial properties fight respiratory infections. Honey coats the throat and has its own antimicrobial effects, creating double-action relief.

SAFETY NOTE: *Not for babies under 1 year due to honey. Generally very safe. Allergic reactions rare but possible.*

SPEARMINT UPSET STOMACH

While peppermint can be too strong for children, spearmint has been the traditional "children's mint" for centuries. Garden-growing mothers always kept a patch just for little tummies.

WHAT YOU'LL NEED:
» 2 tablespoons fresh spearmint (or 1 tablespoon dried)
» 1 cup hot water
» Honey (optional, over 1 year)

HOW TO MAKE IT:
1. Pour hot water over spearmint
2. Cover and steep 5-7 minutes
3. Strain leaves
4. Cool to comfortable temperature
5. Sweeten if desired

USAGE IN TRADITIONS: After meals or for upset stomach: Toddlers 1-2 tablespoons, older children 1/4 to 1/2 cup. Can give every 2-3 hours.

HERBAL INSIGHTS: Spearmint contains gentler volatile oils than peppermint, making it perfect for children. It relieves gas, reduces nausea, and calms digestive spasms without being too cooling or stimulating. The mild flavor appeals to young palates.

SAFETY NOTE: *May cause mild alertness. No known contraindications.*

ROSE HIP IMMUNE GUMMIES

During WWII, British children collected rose hips for the national syrup program. These vitamin C-rich "gummies" kept children healthy when citrus was unavailable.

What You'll Need:
- 1/2 cup rose hip tea (strong)
- 2 tablespoons honey
- 2 tablespoons grass-fed gelatin
- Silicone molds

How to Make It:
1. Make strong rose hip tea
2. Strain carefully (remove all seeds)
3. Heat tea gently, add honey
4. Sprinkle gelatin while whisking
5. Pour into molds quickly
6. Refrigerate until set

Usage in Traditions: 2-4 gummies daily for immune support. Can increase during illness. Store refrigerated up to 1 week.

Herbal Insights: Rose hips provide bioavailable vitamin C that's gentler than synthetic ascorbic acid. The vitamin C supports immune function while the gelatin provides gut-healing proteins. Kids think they're getting candy while receiving powerful immune support.

Safety Note: *Not for children under 2 (choking hazard). High vitamin C may cause loose stools if too many consumed.*

SLIPPERY ELM LOZENGES

Native American children sucked on slippery elm bark like candy. Colonial mothers learned to make lozenges, creating America's first throat drops.

What You'll Need:
- 1/4 cup slippery elm powder
- 2 tablespoons honey
- 1 tablespoon water
- Cinnamon powder (optional)

How to Make It:

1. Mix slippery elm with honey
2. Add water slowly to form thick paste
3. Add pinch of cinnamon if desired
4. Roll into small balls
5. Let dry 24 hours
6. Store in airtight container

USAGE IN TRADITIONS: Let child suck on lozenge for sore throat or cough. Ages 3-6: small pea-sized. Over 6: marble-sized. Maximum 4-6 daily.

HERBAL INSIGHts: Slippery elm creates a protective mucilage coating that soothes irritated throats and suppresses cough reflexes. The coating action lasts longer than liquids, providing sustained relief. The honey adds antimicrobial properties.

SAFETY NOTE: *Choking hazard for young children. Only for ages 3+ who can safely suck lozenges.*

ECHINACEA GLYCERITE

Plains Indian children chewed echinacea roots like gum. Modern herbalists discovered glycerin extraction makes this powerful immune herb palatable for picky young tongues.

WHAT YOU'LL NEED:
» 1/2 cup dried echinacea root
» 1 cup vegetable glycerin
» 1/2 cup distilled water
» Glass jar

HOW TO MAKE IT:
1. Place echinacea in jar
2. Mix glycerin and water
3. Pour over herbs to cover
4. Cap and shake well
5. Store 4-6 weeks, shaking daily
6. Strain and bottle

USAGE IN TRADITIONS: At first sign of illness: 1/4 teaspoon for toddlers, 1/2 teaspoon for older children, 3-4 times daily. Not for prevention.

HERBAL INSIGHTs: Echinacea stimulates immune response when illness threatens. The glycerin extraction is alcohol-free and sweet, making it perfect for children. It's most effective when given at the very first signs of illness.

SAFETY NOTE: *Not for daily prevention. Avoid with autoimmune conditions. Rare allergic reactions in daisy-sensitive children.*

MULLEIN EAR Oil

Mountain mothers picked mullein flowers one by one, infusing them in oil for their children's ear aches. This tedious process created liquid gold for ear pain.

WHAT YOU'LL NEED:
- 1/4 cup mullein flowers
- 1/2 cup olive oil
- 2 garlic cloves (optional)
- Small dropper bottle

HOW TO MAKE IT:
1. Wilt flowers 12 hours to reduce moisture
2. Place in small jar with garlic
3. Cover with olive oil
4. Let infuse 2 weeks in sunny window
5. Strain through coffee filter
6. Bottle in dropper bottle

USAGE IN TRADITIONS: Warm oil to body temperature. Place 2-3 drops in affected ear twice daily. Never use if eardrum is perforated.

HERBAL INSIGHTs: Mullein flowers reduce inflammation and fight infection in the ear canal. Garlic adds antimicrobial properties. The warm oil itself soothes pain while the herbs work on underlying infection. Often provides relief within minutes.

SAFETY NOTE: *Never use with perforated eardrum or drainage. See doctor for severe pain or fever. External ear canal only.*

Seasonal Wellness

Nature provides what we need precisely when we need it. Spring's bitter greens cleanse winter's stagnation, summer's cooling herbs prevent overheating, fall's immune-boosters prepare for cold season, and winter's warming spices maintain circulation through the cold. By aligning our herbal practice with the seasons, we work with natural rhythms rather than against them.

Seasonal Preparation Recipes

SPRING DETOX TEA BLEND

Medieval Europeans did "spring cleaning" for their bodies too, using bitter herbs to "clean the blood" after winter's heavy foods. They were intuitively supporting natural detoxification.

WHAT YOU'LL NEED:
- » 2 tablespoons dandelion root
- » 2 tablespoons burdock root
- » 1 tablespoon red clover blossoms
- » 1 tablespoon nettle leaf
- » 1 teaspoon licorice root

HOW TO MAKE IT:
1. Mix all herbs in bowl
2. Store in airtight container
3. To brew: Use 1 tablespoon blend per cup
4. Steep in boiling water 15 minutes
5. Strain and drink

USAGE IN TRADITIONS: Drink 2-3 cups daily for 2-3 weeks in early spring. Best taken between meals. Can repeat monthly through spring.

HERBAL INSIGHts: This blend supports your liver and kidneys—your body's main detox organs. Dandelion and burdock gently stimulate bile production and elimination pathways. Nettle provides minerals depleted during winter, while red clover supports lymphatic drainage. It's like spring cleaning from the inside out.

SAFETY NOTE: *Not for pregnancy or gallstones. May interact with medications—dandelion is diuretic. Start slowly if prone to detox reactions.*

SUMMER COOLING HIBISCUS DRINK

Egyptians offered hibiscus tea to the sun god Ra to stay cool in the desert. From Jamaica's sorrel to Mexico's agua de jamaica, cultures worldwide use hibiscus to beat the heat.

WHAT YOU'LL NEED:
- 1/2 cup dried hibiscus flowers
- 1/4 cup fresh mint
- 4 cups water
- Honey to taste
- Lime juice

HOW TO MAKE IT:
1. Bring water to boil
2. Remove from heat, add hibiscus
3. Steep 20 minutes
4. Strain, add mint while warm
5. Sweeten and add lime
6. Chill thoroughly

USAGE IN TRADITIONS: Drink throughout hot days. Can consume freely—replaces electrolytes lost through sweating. Serve over ice.

HERBAL INSIGHts: Hibiscus is refrigerant—it actually cools your body temperature. It's also rich in vitamin C and electrolytes, replacing what you lose through perspiration. The tart flavor stimulates salivation, helping you feel less thirsty. This isn't just refreshing—it's functional cooling.

SAFETY NOTE: *May lower blood pressure. Can interact with some medications. Tart flavor may affect tooth enamel—use straw.*

FALL IMMUNE BUILDING SOUP

Chinese grandmothers make medicinal soups when autumn arrives, knowing that building immunity before winter prevents illness. This Western adaptation uses similar principles.

WHAT YOU'LL NEED:
- 6 dried shiitake mushrooms
- 1/4 cup astragalus root slices
- 1 onion, chopped
- 4 garlic cloves
- 2 inches fresh ginger
- 8 cups vegetable or bone broth
- Root vegetables as desired

HOW TO MAKE IT:
1. Soak mushrooms until soft
2. Sauté onion, garlic, ginger
3. Add broth and astragalus
4. Simmer 1 hour
5. Add vegetables, cook until tender
6. Remove astragalus before serving

USAGE IN TRADITIONS: Eat 1-2 bowls several times weekly throughout fall. Can freeze portions. Especially important when others start getting sick.

HERBAL INSIGHTS: This soup is immunomodulating medicine disguised as dinner. Astragalus builds deep immunity, shiitakes contain immune-boosting polysaccharides, while garlic and ginger provide antimicrobial protection. Regular consumption strengthens your defenses before cold season hits.

SAFETY NOTE: *Astragalus not during acute illness—it's for prevention. Remove slices before eating as they're too tough.*

WINTER WARMING CHAI

Indian chai wallahs adjust their spice blends seasonally, adding more warming spices in winter. This wisdom keeps circulation strong when cold would otherwise slow it.

WHAT YOU'LL NEED:

» 2 tablespoons ginger root
» 1 tablespoon cinnamon chips
» 1 teaspoon cardamom pods
» 1 teaspoon black peppercorns
» 1/2 teaspoon cloves
» 4 cups water
» Milk and honey to taste

HOW TO MAKE IT:
1. Combine spices and water
2. Simmer 20 minutes
3. Strain spices
4. Add milk and honey
5. Heat gently
6. Serve hot

USAGE IN TRADITIONS: Drink 1-2 cups daily throughout winter, especially on cold mornings. Warms you from inside out.

HERBAL INSIGHts: These warming spices increase circulation, helping maintain body temperature in cold weather. They also support digestion—important when we tend toward heavier winter foods. The combination provides sustained internal warmth that coffee's quick hit can't match.

SAFETY NOTE: Very warming—reduce if you run hot. May increase blood pressure slightly. Not for acute inflammation.

NETTLE SPRING TONIC

European peasants eagerly awaited spring nettles, knowing they provided minerals lacking in winter's stored foods. "Spring nettle soup" traditions exist across Northern Europe.

WHAT YOU'LL NEED:
» 1 cup fresh nettle tops (or 1/2 cup dried)
» 1 quart boiling water
» Lemon juice
» Sea salt

HOW TO MAKE IT:
1. Place nettles in jar (use gloves if fresh!)
2. Pour boiling water over

3. Cover and steep 4-8 hours
4. Strain, squeezing out liquid
5. Add lemon and salt

USAGE IN TRADITIONS: Drink 2-4 cups daily throughout spring. Can use as base for soups. Refrigerate unused portion.

HERBAL INSIGHts: Nettles are spring's multivitamin—incredibly rich in iron, calcium, magnesium, and trace minerals. They support kidney function (helping clear winter stagnation) while providing nutrients for increased spring activity. The minerals are highly bioavailable in this long-steeped infusion.

SAFETY NOTE: *High in minerals—may affect blood pressure or blood sugar. Fresh plant stings until cooked.*

DANDELION SPRING BITTERS

French farmers made "pissenlit" (wet-the-bed) wine each spring, knowing dandelion's bitter compounds stimulated sluggish winter digestion. The whole plant from root to flower is medicine.

WHAT YOU'LL NEED:
» 1/2 cup fresh dandelion roots and leaves
» 2 cups apple cider vinegar
» 1 tablespoon honey
» Orange peel (optional)

HOW TO MAKE IT:
1. Chop dandelion coarsely
2. Place in jar, cover with vinegar
3. Add honey and orange peel
4. Cap with plastic lid
5. Steep 2-3 weeks
6. Strain and bottle

USAGE IN TRADITIONS: Take 1 tablespoon in water 15 minutes before meals. Can use as salad dressing. Continue throughout spring.

HERBAL INSIGHts: Dandelion's bitter compounds trigger digestive secretions—stomach acid, bile, and enzymes—preparing your system for food. This is especially important in spring when we transition from heavy winter foods to lighter fare. The bitters also support liver detoxification.

Safety Note: *Avoid with gallstones or bile duct obstruction. May increase stomach acid.*

PEPPERMINT SUMMER COOLER

Moroccan mint tea in the Sahara, mojitos in Cuba, mint juleps in the American South—hot climates worldwide use mint to cool down. It's paradoxically warming yet cooling.

What You'll Need:
- 1/2 cup fresh peppermint
- 1/4 cup fresh spearmint
- 4 cups hot water
- Honey and lemon
- Ice

How to Make It:
1. Pour hot water over mints
2. Steep covered 15 minutes
3. Strain and add honey/lemon
4. Chill completely
5. Serve over ice
6. Garnish with fresh mint

Usage in Traditions: Drink freely on hot days. Can spray on skin for cooling. Especially refreshing mid-afternoon.

Herbal Insights: Menthol in peppermint triggers cold receptors, making you feel cooler without actually lowering body temperature. It also promotes sweating—your body's natural cooling system. The aromatic compounds provide mental refreshment too.

Safety Note: *May worsen heartburn in some. Very cooling—don't overdo if you tend toward cold.*

ROSE HIP FALL SYRUP

Scandinavian children gather rose hips after first frost for winter syrup. This tradition ensures vitamin C stores before the long, dark winter—ancient wisdom preventing scurvy.

WHAT YOU'LL NEED:
» 2 cups fresh rose hips
» 3 cups water
» 1 cup honey
» Cinnamon stick

HOW TO MAKE IT:
1. Simmer rose hips in water 30 minutes
2. Mash and strain carefully
3. Return liquid to pot
4. Add honey and cinnamon
5. Simmer until syrupy
6. Bottle and refrigerate

USAGE IN TRADITIONS: Take 1 tablespoon daily for prevention. Increase to 3 times daily at first sign of illness. Children love it on pancakes.

HERBAL INSIGHTS: Rose hips contain more vitamin C than citrus, plus bioflavonoids that enhance absorption. Making syrup in fall ensures you have immune support ready before cold season. The vitamin C is heat-stable when processed correctly.

SAFETY NOTE: *High vitamin C may cause loose stools. Seeds are irritating—strain well.*

GINGER WINTER TEA

Chinese doctors prescribed ginger tea to "kindle digestive fire" in winter. Vikings chewed ginger before battle to warm their blood—different battle, same principle.

WHAT YOU'LL NEED:
» 3 inch fresh ginger root
» 4 cups water
» Honey and lemon
» Pinch cayenne (optional)

HOW TO MAKE IT:
1. Slice ginger thinly
2. Simmer in water 20 minutes
3. Strain ginger
4. Add honey, lemon, cayenne

5. Drink hot

USAGE IN TRADITIONS: Drink 1-2 cups daily in winter, especially morning. Extra beneficial before going out in cold.

HERBAL INSIGHts: Ginger is thermogenic—it actually raises body temperature by increasing metabolism and circulation. It also supports winter digestion when we eat heavier foods. The warming effect lasts hours, unlike coffee's quick spike.

SAFETY NOTE: *Very warming—reduce if you feel too hot. May increase blood pressure slightly. Can interact with blood thinners.*

CLEAVERS LYMPH CLEANSE

Country children called cleavers "sticky willy" and threw them at each other. Wise women gathered the same sticky plant for spring lymphatic cleansing—nature's velcro is also nature's lymph tonic.

WHAT YOU'LL NEED:
- 1 cup fresh cleavers
- 2 cups cool water
- Lemon juice

HOW TO MAKE IT:
1. Chop cleavers coarsely
2. Cover with cool water
3. Let sit overnight
4. Strain in morning
5. Add lemon juice
6. Drink immediately

USAGE IN TRADITIONS: Drink 1 cup each morning for 2-3 weeks in spring. Best on empty stomach. Can also juice fresh plant.

HERBAL INSIGHts: Cleavers specifically supports lymphatic drainage, helping clear the cellular waste that accumulates over winter. It's also mildly diuretic, supporting kidney function. This gentle cleansing helps reduce spring sluggishness and puffiness.

SAFETY NOTE: *Mildly diuretic—stay hydrated. May interact with diuretic medications.*

ELDER FLOWER SUMMER COLD TEA

European grandmothers knew summer colds were the worst—you're already hot and then fever hits. Elder flower tea cools fever while fighting the virus—perfect for out-of-season illness.

What You'll Need:
» 3 tablespoons dried elder flowers
» 1 tablespoon peppermint
» 1 tablespoon yarrow
» 2 cups boiling water

How to Make It:
1. Combine herbs in teapot
2. Pour boiling water over
3. Cover and steep 15 minutes
4. Strain herbs
5. Can serve hot or cooled

Usage in Traditions: Drink hot to promote sweating for fever. Drink cool for summer cold without fever. Take frequently until symptoms resolve.

Herbal Insights: Elder flower promotes sweating to break fever while having antiviral properties. Combined with cooling peppermint and fever-managing yarrow, it addresses summer colds perfectly—cooling the heat while fighting infection.

Safety Note: *Very safe. Promotes sweating—stay hydrated. Elder flowers different from elderberries.*

ASTRAGALUS FALL PREVENTION

Chinese families add astragalus to fall soups, knowing it builds "wei qi" (defensive energy) before winter. This preventive approach keeps families healthy through cold season.

What You'll Need:
» 1/4 cup astragalus root slices
» 4 cups water
» Goji berries (optional)
» Honey to taste

How to Make It:
1. Simmer astragalus in water 45 minutes
2. Add goji berries last 10 minutes
3. Strain out astragalus
4. Sweeten with honey
5. Drink warm

Usage in Traditions: Drink 1 cup daily throughout fall. Can use liquid as base for soups. Not during acute illness.

Herbal Insights: Astragalus is an immune modulator—it trains your immune system to respond appropriately to threats. Taking it preventively in fall builds resilience for winter challenges. It increases production of immune cells while reducing inflammatory responses.

Safety Note: *For prevention only—not during acute illness. May interact with immunosuppressants.*

CINNAMON WINTER CIRCULATION

Medieval spice traders risked their lives for cinnamon, valued for its warming properties. Those who could afford it added cinnamon to wine to survive cold castles.

What You'll Need:
- 2 cinnamon sticks
- 1 teaspoon whole cloves
- 1 tablespoon dried orange peel
- 2 cups water
- Honey and brandy (optional)

How to Make It:
1. Combine spices and water
2. Simmer gently 15 minutes
3. Steep covered 10 more minutes
4. Strain spices
5. Add honey and splash of brandy
6. Serve warm

Usage in Traditions: Drink before going out in cold or when extremities are cold. Especially good for people with poor circulation.

HERBAL INSIGHTS: Cinnamon dilates blood vessels, improving circulation to extremities. Combined with cloves (another warming spice), it creates sustained warmth. This isn't just perception—these spices actually increase peripheral blood flow, warming hands and feet.

SAFETY NOTE: *Can lower blood sugar—monitor if diabetic. Very warming—not for hot constitutions. Cassia cinnamon high in coumarin.*

VIOLET SPRING SYRUP

Victorian ladies made violet syrup for spring garden parties. Beyond its lovely color, they intuitively used a powerful lymphatic herb when bodies needed spring cleansing.

WHAT YOU'LL NEED:
- 2 cups fresh violet flowers
- 2 cups boiling water
- 2 cups sugar or honey
- Lemon juice

HOW TO MAKE IT:
1. Pour boiling water over violets
2. Cover and steep overnight
3. Strain, pressing flowers
4. Add equal amount sugar/honey
5. Add lemon juice (turns purple!)
6. Simmer until syrupy

USAGE IN TRADITIONS: Take 1 tablespoon daily as spring tonic. Can add to water or tea. Children love it on pancakes.

HERBAL INSIGHTS: Violets have special affinity for the lymphatic system, helping move stagnant lymph accumulated over winter. The flowers contain mucilage that soothes respiratory passages.

SAFETY NOTE: *Use only sweet violets (Viola odorata) or wild violets. Some violet species are toxic.*

FOUR THIEVES VINEGAR

Legend says four thieves robbed plague victims without getting sick, protected by this herbal vinegar. When caught, they traded the recipe for their freedom. True or not, it works!

WHAT YOU'LL NEED:
- 1/4 cup each: sage, rosemary, thyme, lavender
- 8 garlic cloves
- 4 cups apple cider vinegar
- 1 tablespoon black peppercorns

HOW TO MAKE IT:
1. Place all herbs in jar
2. Cover with vinegar
3. Use plastic lid (vinegar corrodes metal)
4. Steep 4-6 weeks
5. Strain and bottle
6. Label clearly

USAGE IN TRADITIONS: Take 1 tablespoon in water daily during illness outbreaks. Can use as salad dressing or add to bath.

HERBAL INSIGHTS: Every ingredient is powerfully antimicrobial. The combination creates broad-spectrum protection against bacteria, viruses, and fungi. Used internally, it boosts immunity. Used externally, it can disinfect surfaces. This medieval hand sanitizer still outperforms many modern versions.

SAFETY NOTE: *Very strong—dilute before use. May interact with medications due to garlic. Not for people with acid reflux.*

www.ingramcontent.com/pod-product-compliance
Lightning Source LLC
Chambersburg PA
CBHW020542030426
42337CB00013B/952